SLOW SEX SECRETS

Lessons from the Master Masseur

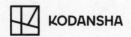

SLOW SEX SECRETS

Lessons from the Master Masseur

Adam Tokunaga

Translated by Marc Adler

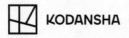 KODANSHA

Slow Sex Secrets: Lessons from the Master Masseur
A VERTICAL Book

Production: Tomoe Tsutsumi

English language version produced by Kodansha USA Publishing, LLC, 2023.

Originally published in Japan as *Surou Sekkusu Jissen Nyuumon* by Kodansha, Ltd., Tokyo, 2006.

Previously issued in English in hardvocer in 2008.

ISBN 978-1-64729-323-9

Printed in the United States of America

First Paperback Edition

Kodansha USA Publishing, LLC
451 Park Avenue South, 7th Floor
New York, NY 10016
www.kodansha.us

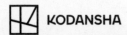 KODANSHA

TABLE OF CONTENTS

SLOW SEX SECRETS

Lessons from the Master Masseur

Chapter One
Modern Society and Authentic Sex

The "Crime and Punishment" of Men who Focus on Immediate Gratification

You want to see a woman naked. You want to touch her body. You want her to give you oral sex. You want to penetrate her. You want to orgasm. You'd even like to make her orgasm, if possible.

That, in a few words, sums up the typical man's motivations when it comes to sex. Notice anything strange about that list? That's right—every item is an immediate pleasure. Men's focus on orgasm, in particular, is second-to-none. We have sex to achieve orgasm—that is what modern sex is all about for men.

You might be thinking that there's nothing unnatural about that, but the fact is that this selfish, single-minded focus on the momentary pleasure of orgasm makes sex boring. For a young couple who are just learning the pleasures of sex, simply enjoying the physical intimacy of each other's bodies is happiness enough. When you're still learning how it all works, your partner accepts your vigorous exertions, even if all you're concentrating on is your own desire to reach orgasm. However, once you become older, and have more experience, your skills must mature along with the rest of your personality.

We all start out as beginners with nothing more to guide us than our libido and curiosity about the other sex. As you fumble through your first experiences, however, you acquire a few techniques and a certain amount of expertise. You are now at the intermediate level, where you experiment with your fingers, tongue, and penis to see if you can make your partner reach orgasm. As you further polish your technique, you begin to connect your love for your partner with her sexuality and realize that true happiness lies in making your partner feel pleasure. Thus, step by step, you reach a more advanced level.

Or at least that's how it should be. It's what it means for a man to become a mature adult, reaching a higher plane of emotional and sexual awareness. Men today, however, never seem to lose their blinkered focus on their own orgasm, no matter how old they get. Just look at how immature so many young men are today, even after they are no longer considered "minors" under the law. If their sexual immaturity is on par with the social immaturity that's been observed in so many of them, then we really have something to be worried about.

Sex is fun—sex, that is, that focuses on caressing. But if sex consists of nothing more than the bare minimum of caressing during foreplay, and then the old one-two of "penetration→orgasm," it's going to be impossible to bring out the latent potential of the countless erogenous zones all over a woman's body. It's a crime for a man not to be able to make a woman reach orgasm, and the punishment for this crime is that you'll never see the true beauty of the woman you love.

Time is of the Essence

Modern society has reduced sex to its most primitive form—a simple act of reproduction, characterized first and foremost by speed. When I surveyed the male students at "Adam," the sex school I run, I found that they spend, on average, fifteen minutes on foreplay, and a mere five minutes from penetration to orgasm. In other words, the average amount of time they spend during sex, from foreplay to orgasm, is twenty minutes. I've heard basically the same from many women (in the form of complaints, mind you)—fifteen minutes of foreplay, five minutes of penetration. This seems to be the average amount of time required for sex in today's world.

Sure, if you're only interested in fertilizing an ovum, then who cares how much time it takes? But the fact is that the majority of people having sex take pains to *avoid* pregnancy. And since that's the case, that average of twenty minutes looks more like a symptom of male impatience to reach orgasm than the outcome of a reproductive act. The truth is that what we call "sex" today is really nothing more than a woman allowing a man to use her body for him to reach orgasm.

The three biggest sexual complaints women have are: their partner reaching orgasm too quickly, unimaginative sex, and a lack of foreplay. Sex that only lasts twenty minutes is going to fulfill all three of those conditions perfectly.

When the conversation turns to the topic of sex, men indicate an interest in questions of "technique," while women tend to focus on "love." Both sides lose sight of the importance of time. The idea that you can satisfy a woman as long as you master certain techniques is as mistaken as a woman's idea that she will enjoy sex as long as she truly loves her partner. Technique and love are, of course, important elements in pleasurable sex, but they are not the only elements. As with many things, true sex requires dedication. To get the most out of sexual techniques and to experience true love, you have to put in a minimum amount of time. Naturally, the minimum time required is most emphatically not twenty minutes.

The reason I use the term "Slow Sex" and focus a spotlight on sex in modern society is that I want people to correct this mistaken understanding of how long it takes to have sex.

"Slow sex" is more than simply a call for people to lengthen the amount of time they have sex, although many of the problems—including the ones that you probably face—could be solved just by turning that twenty minutes into thirty minutes, and that thirty minutes into an hour. In other words, if you are willing to spend more time caressing a woman's body, you will be able to give her pleasure, without recourse to fancy techniques. The key here is "time."

The Spread of "Junk Sex"

Let's take a closer look at this male-focused, orgasm-obsessed, twenty-minute sex—truly the sexual equivalent of junk food—which has unfortunately become the norm in our society. It's no surprise that many women complain of never having experienced orgasm, and that while they may love their partners, their sex lives leave something to be desired. Of course, at least they're complaining. The fact is that more and more women say they shy away from sex, would rather not have sex, and even dislike sex. Sex, one of the greatest pleasures known to humankind—and women are saying they don't want to have anything to do with it! The only explanation is that women view sex negatively, feel an aversion towards it, and even give up on it altogether out of an instinct to protect themselves from the worry, stress, and pain created by male-centered sex. Cultural manifestations of this can be seen in movies and TV shows that idealize pure, romantic love, unsullied by sexual relations.

There are two main factors that have turned modern sex into "junk sex." One is the immature desire of men who haven't become fully formed adults to penetrate their partner as soon as possible and to reach orgasm as soon as possible. The other is the fact that women's advancing place in society has meant that many women have less free time. Ironically, this unfortunate coincidence of men's desire to reach orgasm quickly and women's desire to get it over with quickly has accelerated the transformation of sex into junk sex.

Naturally, the fundamental problem is men's immature desire for sex that focuses solely on them and their orgasm. After all, if sex were more pleasurable for women, they wouldn't want it to be over so quickly.

This unfortunate coincidence is the start of an even greater tragedy. Namely, men's desire for immediate orgasm has created the same desire in women. It is only natural for a woman to want to reach orgasm, but there is no way that a woman can achieve satisfaction or pleasure in a mere twenty minutes of foreplay and penetration. Junk sex reduces what should be an act that is pleasurable, that deepens the partners' love for one another, and that even makes people feel happy to be alive, into something that is greedy, selfish, and guided by raw egotism.

No matter how boring sex becomes, no matter how worthless it is made, however, men still achieve the pleasure of their own orgasm. This is the biggest factor blinding men to the mistake they are making. As it becomes more prevalent, junk sex is creating a gap between men, who experience at least a small amount of pleasure, and women, who experience absolutely no pleasure. Men must wake up to the reality that the more they engage in sex that focuses solely on their own orgasm, the more dissatisfied their partners will become.

As a man, I always assumed that the fault for making sex boring and uninspiring lay with men themselves. It was glaringly obvious (to me) that women who complained that they could not achieve orgasm were the victims of men who didn't care about their partner's sexuality. After speaking with many women, however, my thinking in this area has evolved. With the prevalence of junk sex today, it is becoming clearer and clearer that even women have fallen prey to the junk sex idea of how long sex should last. Proof of this can be found in the fact that there are women who want to skip lengthy foreplay and get right to the immediate gratification of orgasm, despite the fact that they simply require much more time than men to experience true pleasure, due to their physiological makeup. I cannot help but feel an impending sense of crisis before the saddening incongruity of women—ostensibly the victims of modern junk sex—themselves becoming accomplices.

Immature Sex Ruins Love

Whether love comes before sex or sex before love is a perennial topic of articles in women's magazines, but endless analysis that never seems to reach any conclusion frankly turns me off. For the most part, the debate begins by positing that "men can have sex without experiencing love," which is countered—at length—with something along the lines of "sex with love is better." Women are then given the almost Victorian advice that they should not have sex with a man right away, "no matter how much you like him." But if you think the man's going to be kept waiting, you're wrong, because in order to make sure they get their man, women are also given tips for bagging the guy on the spot, "casually putting your hand on his knee" at a party, etc. The advice is contradictory, to say the least. Finally, women are told to "act with the awareness that you are an adult woman," which is another recent common theme—personal responsibility and all that—but that's it.

You can only wonder at the level of maturity of the writer or editor who puts together this kind of article.

Women are certainly a mystery to men, but it goes both ways. It's no excuse for adults to treat the subject of how sex and love are interrelated as though it were the sterile topic of some high-school debate. Asking whether love or sex should "come first" is a pointless, immature waste of time that I am going to put an end to right now. It doesn't matter which comes first, since so much depends on the particular circumstances of each couple. Ethically and morally, there's probably a whole spectrum of opinions on the matter, but whether someone engages in "sex with love" or "sex without love" is a personal choice. Both should be accepted. What we should be focusing on isn't whether love is involved or not, but rather the content of the sex. In other words, what matters is whether the sex is good or not. I cannot stress this enough. To make this point even clearer, I've grouped sexual experience into four types.

1. Good sex with love.
2. Bad sex with love.
3. Good sex without love.
4. Bad sex without love.

Nobody has any complaints about Type #1. That should be obvious. What about Type #3, though? Imagine this situation: "I met someone that I really hit it off with, and we had sex the very same day. It was great." If you have trouble finding a problem with this, that's because there *is* no problem. It's in Type #2 and Type #4 that you'll find problems. Confronted with Type #4, all you can do is shrug, really, since the problem is the result of two consenting adults making their own choices. But what about Type #2? That's the really knotty situation. "I had sex with someone I'm in love with, but it was no good." The common reaction (among both sexes) when confronted with this situation is to say, "Maybe we don't love each other enough" or "does he/she really love me?" In other words, "love" gets the blame for sex that isn't good.

This is a huge mistake. Love is important, but its importance can be exaggerated. No amount of love can overcome a lack of knowledge about sexuality and sexual techniques that can make sex better. Closing your eyes to this self-evident correlation of cause and effect and trying to find the solution in "love" is a kind of willful ignorance that creates emotional stress and walls between couples and can even eat away at whatever true love did exist before a couple started having sex.

In other words, bad sex can ruin love.

If, for whatever sad reason, sex brings nothing but psychological pain and physical discomfort, a young couple can simply break up and reset themselves, as it were. For a married couple, though, bad sex can be tragic. Boring sex leads to sex-as-duty, which really kills all the enjoyment in the act. I have seen more than my fair share of married couples for whom sex, instead of bringing pleasure and intimacy, winds up becoming a source of stress; naturally, this causes them to stop having sex altogether. Is it really that incomprehensible if a woman looks outside her marriage for someone who can give her pleasure? Ironically, all she's looking for from extramarital partners is satisfying sex, so it's easier to achieve a kind of ideal sexual communication with them. I believe this is one reason for the rise in extramarital affairs. Why can't couples in love achieve this kind of simple communication? The irony is almost too great to bear.

Nobody is born knowing how to have great sex. Just as couples who are in love grow fonder of each other over time and mature together, sex is something that both partners must nurture. Everyone starts out inexperienced in the area of technique, but even if you can't give a woman the kind of pleasure she wants, you can slowly learn where to caress her, how much pressure to apply, and so on, as long as you are considerate and have a sincere desire to please her. Everyone naturally acquires a certain amount of technique and expertise, even without a how-to book like this one. There are nevertheless more and more couples who have trouble overcoming the doubts and worries typical of the initial stages of sexual experience. I can't help thinking that there are more and more people today who simply lack the feelings of consideration and care that are a natural part of romantic relationships. Beyond their ignorance about sex and lack of caressing technique, modern men and women simply lack maturity.

In contrast, the Slow Sex that I propose will, if performed correctly, make sex great for everyone, because it's not some rarified theory that reveals the true nature of love (or whatever), but rather a concrete method for helping people regain that joyful feeling of being alive by experiencing the very real happiness of pleasure with their minds and bodies.

I want you, my male readers, to discover through good sex how different women's bodies are from your own, as well as the differences in how they feel pleasure and where they feel pleasure, and also the differences in their attitudes and sensibilities. This will lead you to a deeper understanding of women and translate into a natural wellspring of warm feelings for your girlfriends or wives.

In a word, you will learn hidden truths that were obscured by your past sexual experience, which was focused solely on penetration and orgasm.

Men's Mistaken Belief that "More Friction = More Pleasure"

I hear lots of complaints from women, but recently the most common one has been that it hurts when men rub their clitoris. Guided by their own experience with masturbation, men mistakenly believe that the greater the friction, the more pleasure their partner will feel. Men tend to use too much force in their caressing anyway, and this is true when they rub their partner's clitoris, which is the most sensitive part of her body. You stimulate the clitoris by moving your fingers over it, right? The fundamental rule when doing this, however, is "gently does it." A woman feels no pleasure if you start rubbing her clitoris with your fingers all of a sudden. This has the effect of dampening her reaction. A man who doesn't understand the "gently does it" rule will try to make up for the diminished reaction from his partner by rubbing her clitoris more aggressively, believing "more friction = more pleasure." The result is generally discomfort for the woman, not pleasure, although in order to avoid spoiling the mood, she often won't say anything and simply put up with it. Sadly, the man mistakes the look on his partner's face—furrowed brow, mouth closed tight—as a sign of pleasure, instead of an expression of enduring pain, which is what it actually is. Misreading his partner's expression in this way causes the man to rub her clitoris even more aggressively. It's a common vicious circle.

Before I present the right way to rub a woman's clitoris, however, let's take a look at the fundamentals of the action. Whether you're stimulating your partner's clitoris with your fingers or with your tongue, the fundamental rule is: "gently does it." A good rule of thumb is to reduce the force to one-fifth, or even one-tenth, of the force you normally use. Stimulation that is almost teasingly gentle is just right. And don't stop that gentle rubbing. Just because your partner has started to feel something doesn't mean you should rub harder. You may think that the basic rule is to start gently, and then gradually increase the force, but nothing could be further from the truth. The right way to stimulate the clitoris is "gently does it, from start to finish." The only time you should move your tongue or fingers faster is right before your partner is about to climax. Keeping up a very gentle touch may in certain cases lengthen the amount of time it takes for your partner to reach orgasm, but there's nothing wrong with that. Your primary goal isn't to give her an orgasm, after all. Your goal should be to give her a deeper kind of pleasure for a longer period of time. Orgasm is simply a result of this process. Indeed, the orgasm your partner experiences as a result of a longer, more intense session will be an earth-shattering thing, worlds apart from the more subdued orgasm she would experience otherwise.

The Proper Way to Stimulate a Clitoris

Let's take a look at the right way to stimulate a clitoris, then.

What a lot of men don't know is that the first thing you have to do before stimulating the clitoris is to "pull back the hood." To stimulate this very small erogenous zone accurately, you have to expose the clitoris completely by pulling back the hood of flesh that covers it. Start by having your partner lie on her back, and position yourself next to her. If you're right-handed, you'll probably be better off to your partner's right side.

For the following explanation, we'll assume you are right-handed.

First, pull back the hood with your left hand. To do this, you hold the clitoris between your index and middle fingers, and then spread your fingers, pulling the flesh back, and then move your fingers up about an inch in the direction of your partner's bellybutton. The clitoris should now be exposed.

Now let's look at what to do with your other fingers. With your left hand pulling back the hood of the clitoris, place your right hand on your partner's thigh, with the soft, fleshy side of your palm (below your little finger) resting on the skin. It is important to keep your hand still so that you can provide steady, continuous stimulation with your fingers. Very gently, rub the clitoris by moving your middle finger up and down, moving your wrist in a back-and-forth motion, never letting the side of your hand leave your partner's thigh. Vary the speed with which your finger moves over the clitoris from bottom to top, visualizing the stimulation the whole time.

At first you should look to make sure your finger is accurately stimulating the tip of the clitoris. Sloppiness will ruin everything. Keep checking until your finger gets a feel for the right position.

The Tragedy of Media Influence

We live in an online world, and the importance of being "media literate" is declared from every corner.

"Media literacy," of course, means understanding what defines the media, and knowing how to choose and use only what's relevant to you from the flood of information. The same applies to information about sex, since there is an ocean of misinformation on the subject. The most significant amount of misinformation surrounds the G-spot.

I doubt there's a man alive today who hasn't heard of the G-spot. Unfortunately, about all most men really know about it is that it's the name of an erogenous zone. You, dear reader, are probably not an exception. In all likelihood, you've heard the name, but aren't sure of where it exactly is or how to stimulate it. You've probably read sensationalized stories in men's magazines about the "amazing spot" that causes "female ejaculation," accompanied by misleading diagrams of where it is and how to reach it, and error-riddled descriptions of how to stimulate it. You wonder whether the authors of such articles have actually made a woman orgasm by stimulating her G-spot.

I must also put in a word about the damage done by porn. Not too long ago there was a brief boom in movies showing women squirting liquid as they ejaculated, and this seems to have become pretty standard fare these days—so standard, in fact, that you might actually think that all women can do this. In my experience, however, maybe two or three out of a hundred women ejaculate during sex—that is, have the physiological makeup that permits them actually to ejaculate. Even if they can, such women don't always ejaculate, either. A lot depends on how they are feeling that day, their partner's technique, and other factors. Furthermore, the fact that they ejaculate doesn't necessarily mean it gives them pleasure. I've heard many pornographic actresses complain that not only does it not feel good, they actually feel a measure of discomfort; they do it anyway because "it's part of the job." Of course, this only points to the high level of technique mastered by the male actors they perform with, for whom sex is a vocation, after all. You should not try this at home on your wives or girlfriends. In my view, anybody who forces a woman to ejaculate shouldn't be having sex.

Still, there is no doubt that the G-spot is an amazing erogenous zone. If you can stimulate it accurately, using the right method, in the right location, you'll be able to give your partner an unparalleled sensation, totally different from the pleasure she feels when penetrated or when having her clitoris stimulated.

Chapter Four gives a detailed discussion of how to stimulate the G-spot correctly, so please read it and take your partner on a journey to a land of pleasure she has never experienced before.

Penis Worship is a One-Way Street

Too many men believe that sex is nothing more than inserting their penis into their partner's vagina. Men who fall prey to this kind of penis worship labor under the misconception that penetrating as soon as possible and pumping away is the secret to giving a woman pleasure. A corollary to this belief is that the larger the penis, the more pleasure a woman feels, since after all, for such men, their penis is the only tool they have in sex. Needless to say, they're wrong.

The fact is that most men penetrate their partner too quickly. Far from feeling pleasure, women experience pain if they are penetrated before they are ready. Men typically think that they can insert their penis as soon as their partner's vagina is lubricated. This is also wrong. In one case I'm familiar with, a woman was able to get so lubricated that the bed sheets were sopping wet, even though she was clinically frigid. Granted, this is a pretty extreme case, but the point is that some women secrete lubricant automatically when they are psychologically aroused. In other words, it's not true that a woman is ready to be penetrated just because she is lubricated. The question, then, is when *should* you initiate penetration? All I can say here is that you simply need to gauge the level of her sensual readiness. The most obvious sign that it's okay to penetrate your partner is when she begs you to (obviously). A high-level technique would be to tease your partner by not penetrating her even after she's begging for it, but that's for a later discussion.

Next, let's take a look at that piston-like thrusting that most men perform as soon as they have initiated penetration. At this point, many women say something like, "Wait. Slow down." The reason is this. Vaginas are designed to expand and contract. When a penis is inserted, the vagina adapts its shape to fit the size and shape of the penis, and remembers that size and shape. This is the part of the preparation the vagina goes through in order to be able to feel pleasure, and this proceeds most efficiently when the penis is still. What this means is that if you start pumping away as soon as you enter your partner, her vagina (and her frame of mind) can't achieve the kind of stability required to feel pleasure.

In other words, the best thing to do in order to help your partner achieve a vaginal orgasm is not to start thrusting as soon as you penetrate her, but rather to enter her and then keep still for a while. In fact, keeping still is an effective technique not just immediately after penetration, but also every once in a while during sex, since your partner's sensitivity increases after each pause. It's a very simple technique, so give it a try.

All right, lastly to the question of size. To a greater or lesser extent, all men would like to have a large penis. The idea is that the bigger your penis is, the more pleasure you can give your partner. In reality, this is just a self-serving illusion created by the desire to have a large penis. Even with an average-sized penis, rapid penetration and over-eager thrusting can cause a woman pain, so you can imagine the discomfort felt by a woman put through the same with a larger-than-average penis. It doesn't take a genius to figure that one out.

If you have an impressively large penis, you are undoubtedly very proud of it. Your sexual activity is probably marked by a healthy self-confidence. This can be a trap, however. Men who fall prey to this kind of penis worship, who overestimate the role of the penis, tend to believe that a large penis is a blank check to do whatever they want. The truth is they are only able to give their partner awkward, unskilled sex.

We've all heard stories about a man who slept with a knock-out only to find the sex unsatisfying. A woman with stunning looks can get any man she wants without lifting a finger. The result is that the totality of her sexual technique consists of simply lying there. The same is true for very handsome men, and my own research has shown that there is a striking tendency among men with large penises to do nothing beyond the bare minimum during sex. Such men care only for their own narcissistic needs, ignorant of the fact that they are not satisfying their partners' sexual needs and indeed might be causing them physical discomfort and even psychological pain.

On the other hand, men who lack confidence in their looks or their penises go the extra mile to compensate for those perceived shortcomings. It's a kind of survival instinct, I think, and it's lacking in men who have large penises because they repeat the same mistakes over and over without ever taking the effort to improve their technique. Penis worship founded on a belief that "all you need is a large penis to make a woman happy" is as foolish as the money-worshipping credo that "all you need is money to get everything you want."

Do not fall into the trap of penis worship. Your hands, infinitely more dexterous than your penis, are what will lead your partner to ecstasy. Your fingers, with their finely tuned sense of touch, are what transport the female body to a world of more profound pleasure. Never forget that the old stand-by, the penis, can only come into its own after your fingers have laid the groundwork.

Problem Position

One of the biggest complaints I hear from women is that their partners finish too quickly. There are sexologists who argue that "it's not premature ejaculation as long as you satisfy your partner, even if the sex only lasts a minute," but defining premature ejaculation this way is just moving the goal posts. It's like sexual harassment: no matter how you spin it, the moment the other party experiences discomfort or dissatisfaction, it's a crime. It's simply not possible for a woman to experience satisfaction in just one minute, due to the way her sexual organs are designed. If you're ever with a woman who says she's satisfied after just one minute of sex, rest assured that you're hearing a very generous lie. Don't let the kindness of women or generous definitions of premature ejaculation go to your head. Some statistics say that up to half of all men experience premature ejaculation, but there's no strength in these numbers—do not let them reassure you. Overcoming premature ejaculation is vital to making sex more enjoyable.

So, why does premature ejaculation occur? The lack of resistance of the penis is the biggest factor, naturally, but what's interesting is that the most common sexual position, the so-called "missionary position," actually includes factors that can cause men to ejaculate prematurely. As a matter of fact, of the many positions available, the missionary position is the one that leads to the fastest ejaculation.

Let's analyze this in detail. In the missionary position, the man's body assumes a forward-leaning attitude. The male ejaculatory mechanism is closely linked with the sympathetic and parasympathetic nervous systems, which are part of the human autonomic nervous system. When the body is leaning forward the sympathetic nervous system, which causes heightened sensitivity in the nerves, takes precedence, causing greater sensitivity in the friction between the penis and the vagina. Added to this is the fact that in this position there is greater freedom for pelvic thrusting, making it easy to enter a sexual "full-attack" mode. In this position, men who lack confidence in their ability to hold out invariably ejaculate in very little time, and this is hardly surprising. Indeed, the missionary may well be called the "immediate-ejaculation position," so men who tend towards premature release should avoid starting out in it.

Conversely, if the man is lying face-up, holding his partner on top of him, the parasympathetic nervous system comes into play, suppressing his arousal and allowing him to enter a state of greater relaxation. This has the effect of making it harder for him to ejaculate. Just by changing positions, the same man, with the same penis, can dramatically extend his endurance. Knowing this simple fact can allow you to hold out much longer and to share your partner's pleasure that much longer.

Ignorance on this point is a crime. Knowing the facts can make you happier.

Sex Defies Medical Definition

There are, to this day, gynecologists who assert, incorrectly, that the vagina is incapable of sensation. Their thinking is that since there aren't sufficient nerves in the vagina, it is impossible for it to feel anything. This is such a fundamental misconception that it is almost silly to rebut it. The G-spot, for one, is obviously on the A-list of erogenous zones, and that's only the beginning. As I lay out in Chapter Four, I have already discovered other areas, such as the Adam G-spot, the T-spot, and the A-spot, whose amazing powers—beyond that of the G-spot—have been proven in sessions with many women.

The misconception that the vagina is not sensitive probably arises through comparison with the nearby clitoris, which allows women to reach orgasm very easily. In comparison, it is difficult to achieve orgasm through the vagina. What I want to stress here is that the degree of ease with which a woman can achieve orgasm through stimulation of a particular erogenous zone is simply a characteristic of that zone, not a judgment about its sensitivity, which is a separate question altogether. Don't forget—women react very strongly when penetrated.

Besides the vagina and clitoris, women's bodies abound in erogenous zones, each of which is unique in nature. The spectrum of pleasure provided by them is broad, ranging from "strong" and "deep" to "gentle" and "faint." It's similar to the way the same musical instrument can produce different tones and timbres, depending on who plays it, and how. In this sense, the female body is a veritable orchestra of many instruments, and you are the conductor. By understanding the nature of each instrument and bringing out its potential, you can perform a symphony of pleasure on your partner's body. It might be difficult for men, who know only penile pleasure, to fathom the mysteries of the female body, but this is the reality of women's bodies, and the essence of sex for them. I use the metaphor of musical instruments because it is important to use an accurate image in order to understand female sexuality.

I stated above how difficult it can be for women to achieve vaginal orgasm, but that was in the context of penetrative sex. Climax may be difficult to reach for your partner if you simply thrust away, but there are erogenous zones in the vagina that can bring a woman to screaming

orgasm if you are able to provide accurate stimulation
to just the right spot. The best-known is the G-spot. The
vagina becomes a very different place when stimulated by
your fingers instead of your penis. Naturally, the penis has
its strong points, and we mustn't forget that the penis can
give a woman a totally different dimension of pleasure.

The crux of the problem is that men insist on making
their partner orgasm through her vagina. A woman
feels a great deal of pressure as she watches her partner,
sweaty and grimacing, try to bring her to orgasm through
penetration. She feels guilty in the face of her partner's
strenuous exertions—that it's her fault that she can't
orgasm, because she's not sensitive. It's no wonder so
many women have trouble achieving orgasm when you
consider the pressure they feel.

I wrote that women can achieve vaginal orgasm more
easily through manual stimulation than by penetrative
sex, but this is only true if their partner has mastered the
proper technique. Ignorant of this fact and misled by false
information, women are prone to stress and misgivings
about not being able to achieve orgasm, which causes
them to shun sex. The fact is that the vast majority of
women can't achieve vaginal orgasm. It is not true that
women who cannot orgasm through penetrative sex
have less sensitivity. It's a simple matter of individual
difference. When a woman wonders why she can't achieve
vaginal orgasm despite trying so hard, she is an example

of the damage done by penis worship. As the man, it's more important that you create a relaxed mood, with no pressure, for your partner to enjoy sex, rather than try to make her orgasm. If your partner happens to achieve orgasm, then great—that's the ideal attitude.

The Difference between Male-Centeredness and "Taking the Lead"

When an ignorant man gives free rein to his ego and his libido, the result is junk sex. Men lose control when they are stoked by an immediate desire for ejaculation. Sex in essence becomes a form of selfish masturbation whose only goal is ejaculation as they lose all interest in their partner's pleasure or satisfaction. Men often mistake this kind of behavior as "taking the lead" in bed. The historical chauvinism seen in all cultures is expressed in this type of male dominance which blinds men to the true role of sex. These days we're used to the idea of women no longer being treated as an inferior sex. Perhaps the fact that the bedroom is the only place where men can be dominant is spurring junk sex tendencies.

I don't want to cause any misunderstandings, so I'll be clear: in matters of sex, men and women should be equals. Anachronistic views placing men above women do as much to restrict and constrain sex as the commonly held belief that men are the aggressors in sex while women play a compliant role. Neither view will lead to a fuller sexual life. On the other hand, the desire on the part of many women for the man to take the lead is not a contradiction. We cannot deny that, by nature, men display a greater tendency than women to be initiators, just as we cannot deny the difference in the physiological makeup of the sexes—men with their erogenous faculties concentrated in their penis, women with their erogenous zones all over their body, from the top of their head to the tips of their toes.

What I want to focus on here is the division of roles between men and women. I want to sound the alarm against the current, very superficial understanding of this as being nothing more than "man inserts penis into woman, woman receives penis"—in other words, against the view that "taking the lead" means the man does everything.

Ideal sex is when both partners stimulate and arouse each other equally. It's not just the man who should be doing this. The woman should also caress and stimulate her partner, helping him to discover a new self-awareness. That is what sex is all about. For mutual stimulation and arousal to occur, the mechanism in the woman's brain that makes her want to work on the man's body must be activated. For this to happen, however, the man must help his partner get rid of any feelings of shame she has that equate female expressions of sexual desire with notions of immorality, or "sluttiness." You're only truly "taking the lead" when you are able to do all this while showing consideration for your partner's femininity. This is the kind of "manliness" that most women subconsciously desire.

Indeed, sex doesn't start in bed. Creating a relationship in which both partners can talk about sex freely is vital. Think about the difference between relationships that focus on the man's desires, on the one hand, and what it truly means to "take the lead," on the other. There will undoubtedly be much food for thought for most of my readers.

Men, Be Receptive!

Men who are unable to free themselves from the old-fashioned stereotype that the man should be active and the woman passive in fact haven't had enough experience letting a woman minister to them. Most men no doubt enjoy fellatio and receive plenty of attention to their penis, but if that is the only part of their body that has received a woman's caresses, they are certainly missing out. Men can experience greater pleasure than they think.

In other words, both men and women should caress each other's bodies all over. In the previous section

I described that the ideal of sex is achieved through mutual caressing and arousal. This means caressing and stimulating each other to your hearts' content, being a sexual glutton for each other's bodies. Simply imagining it is erotic and pleasurable, isn't it? But to focus only on this visual aspect, though it can induce an out-of-the-ordinary eroticism, is to understand less than half of the true wonder of mutual stimulation and arousal. The pleasure you get from sex is proportionate to the "sexual energy" you put in.

I'll go into "sexual energy" in greater depth in the next chapter, but for now you can simply think of it as "the feeling you get when you are sexually aroused." Men know from experience that a woman becomes more sensitive, the greater her arousal. In scientific terms, an increase in sexual energy means heightened receptivity to stimulus in the brain, the enhanced sensitivity of erogenous zones. Sexual energy is something both men and women have, and feeding off of each other's sexual energy amplifies it.

Through caressing each other, both you and your partner become more receptive to pleasure. You see each other in a state of heightened arousal which further arouses you, magnifying the sexual energy, which in turn makes you more sensitive...and so on. This endless "feedback loop of pleasure" is the gateway to an infinite world of sexual bliss.

Don't worry about understanding the mechanism of

sexual energy for now. Just know that the kind of junk sex whereby the man ejaculates and that's all she wrote doesn't involve the necessary give-and-take that is vital to good sex.

To repeat, the current state of affairs, in which men are too seldom the recipients of their partner's caresses, is a terrible waste. Correctly implemented, Slow Sex can transform the pleasure of an orgasm from a minor tremor to an earth-shattering paroxysm of pleasure.

Chapter Two
Sexual Differences

Women and Sexual Gratification

When a woman derives a lot of pleasure from sex or orgasms easily, people say that her erogenous zones have been "trained." You might tell a friend that your girlfriend was "trained" by her previous lover, who was much older, as a way of explaining why she is so sexually receptive. Or, more locally, you might tell your friend, "The girl I did last night had anal training!" My complaint here is that men tend to think that it's the erogenous zones themselves that are doing the feeling. Naturally, this isn't true; the sensitivity of the skin over an erogenous zone isn't exceptional. The brain is actually doing the feeling. Take vision. We say that we see things with our eyes, but in fact it's only after the object has been perceived by the brain that "seeing" really begins. The eyes are just an aspect of the mechanism of vision, like the lens on a camera.

The same can be said for sexual pleasure and orgasm. When a woman's erogenous zone (i.e., skin) is stimulated, it is the brain that decides whether that stimulus feels good or not, and it is in the brain that pleasure is felt, and orgasm attained.

To repeat: it is in the brain, and not the erogenous zones, that pleasure is experienced. In other words, sex *is* all in the mind, and if you lose sight of this very obvious fact, you're going to have trouble giving your partner pleasure and bringing her to orgasm.

Men generally talk about a woman reacting strongly or weakly to stimulus. Individual differences aside, the level of sensitivity for tactile stimulus of the skin is pretty much the same among all women. In other words, there's no such thing as a woman who is more sensitive to sexual stimulus, on a purely physiological level. Differences in reaction to sexual stimulus and in perceived sensitivity are at bottom psychological differences.

What this means is that men should focus on how to open their partners up mentally—how to make them mentally more sensitive to sexual stimulus.

I want to point out again how stupid junk sex is. If you meet a woman who is "sensitive to sexual stimulus," you are so taken by how receptive she is that you forget to "stimulate her brain," focusing instead on your own pleasure. And if you meet a woman who is not sensitive to sexual stimulus, then you just throw in the towel and forget about the whole thing. In both cases, no effort is made to engage the woman's mind, the result being that 99% of women in the world have never known true feminine sexual pleasure.

When "Frigidity" Becomes the Norm

The orgasm that most women experience today is by far not the upper limit of what women can feel. The fact that women can be heard to say "At least, I came" ironically points to the poverty of sexual practice in modern society. I have met many women in their thirties, forties, and even fifties who have never experienced an orgasm. It's sad, but true. Most of the women who come to my school are worried they are frigid and have to get up the courage to come to me for help—women who have little sexual experience, women who have been subjected to rough sex, verbal abuse, or other trauma at the hands of men. While there are many factors contributing to "frigidity" (itself a potential symptom of other problems), the reason they come to me, afraid they might be frigid, is that they're not enjoying sex with their boyfriends or husbands.

Since you have read this far, you can probably guess that there is in fact nothing wrong with 95% of the women who take our frigidity therapy classes. Women come in gloomy, complaining that they don't feel anything during sex with their partners, wondering if something isn't right with their bodies. I subject them to my "orgasm massage," and they writhe and squirm, arch their backs, tremble with pleasure, and scream and moan like wild animals, slowly sinking into an ocean of orgasm. After the procedure, I tell them that there is nothing wrong with their bodies. Their only problem is their bad luck in not having found the right partner.

That might be painful to hear, but it's my frank opinion and an indisputable fact. Women who have had many sexual partners, women who have been married for decades, women who no longer feel anything at their lovers' touch—for the first time in their lives they all experience the kind of pleasure that makes them happy to be alive when they undergo the procedure I apply. Indeed, many women are so overwhelmed by the experience that they cry. This isn't just empty boasting. If you master the sexual techniques I teach in this book, you too will be able to lead your partner to a world of profound sensuality. You will liberate yourself from the shackles of instant gratification; freed from a focus on your own ejaculation, you'll realize the dream of bringing any woman to orgasm. Which is great not just for your partners, but for you, too.

A lack of real sexual experience prevents most men from imagining ideal sex in all its rich potential. That is why if you want to make any progress you must first have a thorough understanding of the current state of women's sexuality and the female sexual mechanism.

Women are "frigid" when their brains are unable to recognize physical stimulus to their skin as "sexual." There are many methods for bringing this function of the brain to life and helping it mature. The most effective and efficient is to supply precise, continuous stimulus to all the erogenous zones over the entire body. Unfortunately, this is beyond the ability of most men. No one knows less about where a woman's erogenous zones are actually located than the students in my own beginning courses. Armed with nothing more than a vague notion of where the zones are, they apply stimulation where they think they ought to but miss the mark by far. They don't really seem to care, either. This is the golf equivalent of teeing off at the third hole aiming for fifth. There is no way the ball is going to reach the cup. When you see that they don't even realize their blunder, you don't know whether to laugh or to cry.

The next most common factor making women think they are frigid is that women themselves don't really know what it is to reach orgasm. I've heard women say, "I feel pleasure when my partner stimulates my clitoris and nipples, but I don't feel like I've reached orgasm." This problem arises because women don't ejaculate like men do; they lack a visible indication that they have reached orgasm. At what level of pleasure can a woman be said to have achieved orgasm? Women themselves aren't so sure. The fact is that they are indeed achieving orgasm, but they've read so many descriptions (e.g., in erotica) of orgasms involving, say, fainting, that they decide that they must be frigid since they aren't fainting. This irrational ranking of levels of sexual pleasure has a negative effect and can even cause actual frigidity.

This all goes to show how closely a woman's sexual sensitivity is tied up with her mind.

In practice, it is important not to pressure a woman to reach orgasm. Don't even think of asking her if she reached orgasm after having sex: that's pressure. The female orgasm is more complicated than the male orgasm, which is basically just ejaculation. No man worries if he's going to be able to ejaculate, but women do worry—seriously—about whether they will be able to reach orgasm.

The trick to helping your partner reach orgasm is to avoid trying to force it and to stop worrying about whether she did or didn't. It may seem counterintuitive, but you're doing more to help your partner succeed in reaching orgasm by taking off the pressure.

Faking It

According to a survey done by a women's magazine, 80% of adult women have faked an orgasm at least once in their lives. Faking it is impossible for men, since there's physical evidence, but it is starting to become the norm in modern sex for women to fake orgasms.

While there is only one real motivation for a woman to fake an orgasm—namely, because she can't reach orgasm—we can point to two further factors. The first one is mercy. A woman might not want to spoil the mood or injure her partner's pride, so she fakes an orgasm. The hope here is that, even if the woman herself isn't enjoying herself, at least she can help her partner enjoy himself. All we can do, as men, is be grateful for such undeserved consideration.

The other factor is rather more grim. Women sometimes fake orgasms to make the pain stop. They figure that if they fake an orgasm, their partner will stop, because the pain is simply unbearable. It's basically a strategy to get their partner to terminate the discomfort and piston-like thrusting.

Men cannot distinguish between these motivations. Men can't even tell if a woman is faking an orgasm or not. Women are born actresses; men, obsessed as they are with their own ejaculation, don't stand a chance of telling the difference between a real orgasm and a faked one.

Either way, the problem is that most men assume that they are great lovers when their partner fakes an orgasm, when in fact they are simply repeating the same mistakes over and over. Once they see (or rather, think) they've had success with a certain technique, they mistake it for some almighty card and use it forever after that even when their partner begins showing a lessened response, and even when their partner changes.

While I pride myself on the general applicability of the techniques I teach in this book, that doesn't mean they are almighty or somehow perfect. In sex, application is everything. You have to learn the basics of a technique to use as a reference point, making small adjustments while carefully observing your partner's responses. Learning the fundamentals helps you to respond to ever-varying situations; maintaining the flexibility to make small adjustments is where your technique will really shine. This principle applies equally to me, an expert sex technician, as it does to you, reading this book.

Don't be deceived by your partner's fake orgasms.

Women Want It Over Quickly?

I have stated that the fundamental problem confronting sex in the modern age is how little time it takes to have it. It is impossible to give a woman satisfying pleasure if the act, including foreplay, only takes twenty minutes. It is simply impossible for a woman to feel pleasure in twenty minutes.

The blame for this (very short) twenty-minute span lies with men. It's not that men want sex to be over quickly, but they want to ejaculate quickly, and this ejaculation-focused, instinctual sex results in the twenty-minute time frame. I always believed most women wanted "to be loved longer." The facts turned out to be somewhat different.

If I ever tell a female acquaintance that the average length of my sexual sessions is two hours, her reaction is inevitably, "That's way too long," always followed by words along the lines of, "What do you spend two hours doing?" I explain that my partner and I spend the time stimulating each other. The next response is a variation of "My jaw would get sore," "I'd start hurting down there," or "I've never had sex for two hours straight, and I don't think I could handle it."

These women imagine my "two hours" as two solid hours of never-ending fellatio or thrusting. They think that stimulating a man means fellating him and that "sex" means the man banging away at the woman's vagina. Since they don't equate either of those acts with pleasure, they can't fathom what I mean when I say my partner and I "enjoy" ourselves during those two hours.

Each of a woman's erogenous zones creates a different sensation of pleasure. Each of those sensations finds a unique expression in a woman's sensual reaction during sex, which means that you can see different aspects of your partner's sensuality as you stimulate different zones. *That is the essence of sexual pleasure!* There's almost an infinite number of these zones all over a woman's body.

Done right, sex is a thousand times more "fun" than any movie or amusement park. Two hours is barely enough, and it passes in a flash.

But women who don't know how good it can feel don't understand this. It makes sense, since it's one of those things that you have to experience to believe. The saddest thing, however, is the sense you get from many women that they've simply given up on sex altogether. Indeed, many women have sex just to help their partners have a good time. That's why they want it to end so quickly.

Men and women are at heart "horny" animals. The modern dynamic in which men want sex and women look down on men as being "horn dogs" is bad for both men and women.

"Orgasm" and "Experiencing Pleasure"

One of the reasons a surprising number of men and women can't experience pleasure in sex is that they confuse "orgasm" and "pleasure." These are two different things altogether. Even to posit "orgasm" as the natural result of "pleasure" is to understand sex in a very narrow sense.

When I explain this to my students, I use the "glass of water" analogy.

When your body is experiencing pleasure, it is like a

glass gradually filling with water. Orgasm, on the other hand, is the instant when the glass is so brimming with water that it overflows. "Filling up" and "overflowing" are two totally different phenomena.

At the heart of this analogy is sexual energy—the same sexual energy which you produce during sexual excitement and stimulation. "Feeling pleasure" means creating and storing up sexual energy, and "orgasm" is the explosive release of that energy. Both men and women orgasm, but in the case of men, orgasm involves ejaculation. But whether you're a man or a woman, it feels good, doesn't it? Of course it does. But think back on your past sexual experiences. You've probably had so-so orgasms, which weren't very satisfying, and earth-shattering orgasms, which seemed to reconfigure your brain. The difference lies in how much sexual energy you stored up prior to the orgasm.

Depending on your makeup, you can probably reach orgasm in about a minute—stroking your penis if you're a man, or stimulating your clitoris with a vibrator if you're a woman. This is the equivalent of filling the glass with only a little bit of water, then forcing the glass over to empty it. You might experience a bit of pleasure, but nothing like true satisfaction.

Do you see why I distinguish between pleasure and orgasm? The objective of the Slow Sex method is to maximize the total amount of sexual energy you and your partner store up—enjoying mutual stimulation without a thought for the clock. Eventually, your sessions will grow to two and even three hours in length, and it will be effortless. You and your partner will be brimming over with sexual energy, and when you reach that explosive orgasm, it will almost be as an afterthought to your mutual enjoyment and stimulation (the whole point of sex, after all) rather than the attainment of a craved goal.

This is where it gets hard. I used the analogy of a glass filling with water to explain how sexual energy is stored up, but the fact of the matter is that if you, like many people, are used to having "junk sex," then your "sexual vessel" is indeed only the size of a drinking glass. As you practice the Slow Sex method, however, and redirect your aim from "orgasm" to "pleasure," you will be expanding the size of that vessel. They say women have an unlimited capacity to feel pleasure, and they're right; with the application of the proper technique, you can help your partner's vessel grow to the size of a bucket, and from there to the size of an oil drum, and so on. There's literally no limit. Imagine all the sexual energy stored up when your partner's container is the size of a dam. Now imagine all that energy surging forth in an earth-shattering explosion as the dam breaks. Just as there's no comparing a glass and a dam, the explosion of pleasure a woman can experience is something we men will never be able to imagine. Women have this amazing potential, and what's important to remember is that the potential is given to all women equally.

The reason women complain about sex so often is that their partners can't even fill up their "small glasses" with sexual energy. It goes to show how incorrect the techniques and attitudes men have brought to sex have been.

Secret Ejaculation Mechanisms

So, why does ejaculation occur? In this section, I'll discuss the mechanism of ejaculation, which men think they understand but actually don't.

Let's start by considering masturbation. Normally, a man strokes the length of his penis with his hand. The head of the penis is connected to the skin on the shaft at a "seam" behind the head of the penis. The tip of the penis vibrates rhythmically as the skin on the shaft is moved up and down by the stroking motion. This rhythmical stimulus is transmitted to the brain, and after a certain number of repetitions, the brain flips a switch to initiate ejaculation, and thus the man ejaculates.

In the previous section we saw the difference between "orgasm" and "pleasure." Men don't simply ejaculate because they feel good, but rather because the brain flips this switch. In other words, if the "ejaculation switch" goes off when enough sexual energy has been stored up, the ejaculation will be satisfying. If not, then the ejaculation will not be as satisfying.

Most men don't know how to make their penis feel pleasure. Men may not have the untapped wellsprings of pleasure women are born with, but we can still feel intense pleasure the way women do if we work at increasing our sexual energy by enjoying the simple feeling of pleasure itself.

First, you have to make sure you thoroughly understand the mechanism of ejaculation I just described. If you do, you'll become aware of a different way of thrusting your hips during sex.

The problem is that men who are used to junk sex have trouble controlling their desire to ejaculate. Many of my students tell me that even though they understand intellectually that it's better to store up the sexual energy, in practice they get excited when they feel erogenous pleasure and begin wanting to ejaculate right away. Once that happens, they stop caring about anything else and go after that ejaculation.

If you really want to enjoy the feeling of pleasure afforded by sex and achieve more intense sensations, you have to re-educate your junk sex-infused brain and penis. The quickest way to do this is to change the way you masturbate.

The two masturbation techniques I discuss here are

ways of stimulating the head of your penis, which is the most concentrated erogenous zone. These methods do not involve vibrating the tip of the penis rhythmically and therefore don't cause the "ejaculation switch" to flip, thereby allowing you to experience the sensation of your sexual energy building as you enjoy the pleasure over a long period of time.

Before starting, make sure you have some kind of massage oil, like the kind they sell at the Body Shop. Don't use hand lotion. The friction coefficient of massage oil is a much better match for the erogenous sensation of the tip of your penis.

Rolling
1. Apply oil to your penis and to the palm of the hand which will grip the head of your penis.
2. With the hand you don't favor, grip the bottom of your penis, pulling down the skin of the shaft.
3. Grip the head of your penis in the center of your palm, and roll your hand around, so that the palm of your hand circles the head of your penis, rubbing the front, sides, and back of it.
4. Repeat Step 3.

What's important is creating as large an area of contact between your hand and the head of your penis as possible, and that the contact is not lost as you roll your hand. The center of the palm has a pressure point which emits sexual energy, so the sensation of pleasure will grow as the friction and the sexual energy combine.

Squeezing
1. Make a loose circle with the hand you favor.
2. Slide that circle down your penis from the head, slowly and gently rubbing the head until just past the protruding part.
3. Slide the circle up over the head of your penis, making sure not to pull the skin of the shaft up as well.
4. Repeat Steps 2 and 3.

The goal of these masturbation methods is to feel pleasure, but not to ejaculate. They should be performed in a relaxed manner. Suppress the urge to stroke your penis the way you normally do, and if you feel yourself start to ejaculate, stop your hand. Continue for at least fifteen minutes, and you'll experience a surge of pleasure unlike anything you've ever felt through ordinary masturbation, which lasts just a few minutes.

This sensation of sinking into an ocean of pleasure is the sensation you should feel during sex. And since during sex you and your partner are combining your sexual energies, you'll feel like you're floating at the bottom of a vast ocean of pleasure. These masturbation techniques are the entrance to a deeper kind of sensuality than you've known from rapid ejaculation and orgasm.

You'll also be enhancing the endurance of your penis by spending time on these masturbation techniques. If you don't have a lot of confidence in your endurance, these techniques can help you overcome problems of premature ejaculation.

Proper Fingering Technique

The number of women who dread having men manually stimulate their vaginas is growing quickly. The biggest reason is the "squirting" boom in porn movies. Many men imitate the hand movements they see male actors perform on actresses in porn movies in an effort to get their own wives or girlfriends to "squirt" in the same way, and they wind up scratching the vaginal walls, causing bleeding and psychological trauma. You should never stick your fingers into your partner's vagina and move them around violently. It isn't just painful. It's extremely dangerous.

That said, if stimulated right, the vagina can be an amazing erogenous zone. I cover specific techniques in Chapter Four, but right now I'll discuss "proper fingering technique" that works for women who haven't had a lot of experience, who have narrow vaginal openings, or who have experienced some sort of trauma in the past.

Before starting, you need massage oil. From now on, you should always use massage oil during sex. Your partner's vagina does secrete lubricating fluids, but the amount secreted varies from woman to woman, and either way, no woman can keep secreting lubricant endlessly. Even if a woman starts out well lubricated, she might dry out at some point. Remember, the amount of lubrication that a woman is producing is *not* a good barometer of the pleasure she is feeling. In order to stimulate a woman for a long period of time, massage oil is a necessary tool.

Some men use saliva as a substitute for a woman's natural lubricant. If you're one of those men, stop. Saliva dries very quickly, smells bad when it dries, and is a turn off to most women (it is kind of gross, after all).

Now, the proper way to insert your fingers. First, have your partner lie on her back with her legs slightly spread apart. Sit in front of her. You're going to insert your index and middle fingers, but first place the tips of your fingers against the vaginal opening and, with the thumb of your other hand, spread the labia on one side out so as to widen the opening. Insert your fingers about half an inch. Pull the labia on the other side out and then insert your fingers another half-inch. Repeat this until your fingers are all the way in.

What's important is to keep the palm of your hand facing up and to insert your fingers parallel to the vaginal cavity; in other words, straight in, and not at an angle. A lot of men turn their hands as they insert their fingers, in a rotating motion, but this can hurt (and scare) a woman, so never do this.

Women's Bodies are for Loving

I come in contact with a lot of women's bodies as part of my work, and the more I see, the more I'm stunned by the beauty of the female body. I'm not what they call a "boob man"; yet, just the sight of a rise of breasts underneath a piece of clothing gets me excited. I sometimes go to strip bars as part of my research, and I'm always amused by the sight of older men sitting front and center, devouring the young women's bodies with their eyes. You really get a sense that it's ingrained in the male DNA to be mesmerized by the beauty of a woman's curves, by that smooth feel unique to a woman's skin. The desire is as natural as breathing and as inescapable as death.

You're probably nodding your head in agreement as you read this. What many men who don't know how to please a woman sexually aren't aware of, however, is that the beauty of a woman's body increases as it is loved. Your partner's body will show a totally new and more beautiful side of itself—something ordinarily unimaginable—if you stimulate her using correct techniques based on correct information. I can't even count the times I've witnessed the quiet, polite type begin to writhe erotically; the cool, intellectual type to talk so dirty you'd think she was a pro; and the modest marital beauty to enter into a sensual dance. The beauty of the ever-changing female form when it writhes, stretches, and even trembles as a man stimulates it is breathtakingly beautiful. It's something beyond erotic or sexual or even "kinky"—it's almost religious. It's not just the outward form that seems to glow; traditionally female attributes like kindness, sensitivity, considerateness, and the power to heal mature and grow as you stimulate your partner's body.

Only another man can stimulate all the innumerable erogenous zones on a woman's body, which is why I think women were born to be loved. There's no other way to explain the staggering difference in the number of erogenous zones in men's and women's bodies. Good sex is the best way to make a woman even more beautiful, and as a man, it is your mission to flip the switch on your partner's internal mechanism to bring out that beauty.

Common Sense about Caresses

Sex is all in the brain. If a woman's brain heightens her sensitivity to her partner's caresses, all of her body becomes sensitized—her elbows, ankles, shins, even her nostrils! In other words, her entire body becomes one big erogenous zone. I sometimes refer to erogenous zones as "pressure points," but the pressure points on a woman's body far outnumber the ones known to Eastern medicine. There are more erogenous zones scattered over a woman's body than there are stars in the sky.

Okay, so even men with little experience in sex know that there are a lot of erogenous zones on a woman's body. What even women don't know and aren't aware of is that each of them offers a unique sensation. Stimulating a woman's earlobe makes her feel something completely different from stimulating her nose, for example, and the same can be said for fingers and toes, and even the big toe and the little toe. When you stimulate these different areas, your partner's reactions can range from a faint feeling of pleasure that causes a slight gasp or an involuntary movement of the hips, to more visceral sensations that make her moan and scream like an animal. Some pleasures are so intense that she can only arch her back in exquisite silence. I described sex as a symphony of pleasure, and a woman's body really is like an orchestra that is filled with uniquely voiced instruments. The arrangement of the instruments differs from woman to woman, so using the same method to stimulate the same erogenous zone can elicit a totally different reaction.

God has endowed women with bodies entirely different from those of men, who can barely muster a grunt during release.

Sex is filled with variations. Women's erogenous zones bespeak the truth that the definition of good sex is enjoying its kaleidoscopic pleasures. Stimulating the clitoris will give a woman pleasure, but no matter how advanced your technique and how great it feels for the woman, there's a limit to the amount of pleasure she'll get from the same stimulus repeated over and over. As all the different pleasures are transmitted to the brain—the faint sensation of a palm caressed, the soft feel of a breath on her neck, the earth-shaking bliss of her pubic bone vibrating— the rich variations combine to produce a sensual medley greater than the sum of its sequences.

Think about playing a piano. Playing with two hands produces a richer sound than with one hand; if you add the pedals, even greater is the depth and variation. The exact same thing can be said about sex.

Some of you may be saying to yourselves, "Everybody knows that. I don't need someone to tell me that I need to stimulate different parts of my partner's body. I already do that." That may be true, but the problem is how most men do this.

"What's wrong with my technique?" you may ask. Well, it's actually not a question of technique. More to the point is the amount of time spent stimulating each erogenous zone, and the order in which the zones are stimulated.

A question to those of you who "already know all

this": what areas exactly are you stimulating? The answer is probably: "a little bit here, a little bit there." Am I right? If so, then all you're doing is randomly touching those parts of your partner's body that your own desire and curiosity dictate.

If you want to make your partner feel good, the way to maximize her sensitivity and receptivity is to very gently stimulate one erogenous zone for a certain amount of time—generally, three to five minutes. That's how long it takes for water to boil. To be totally honest with you, "a little bit here, a little bit there" is basically meaningless.

The women who attend my school receive focused stimulus to specific parts—the ankle, or the collar bone, for example—and are astounded by the effect. They say things like, "I had no idea it felt so good! I've never had that one place touched for so long." What's this if not proof that most men are guilty of the "little bit here, and there" school of caress?

Next is the order of stimulation. I'll give a brief overview of the actual order we teach at my school.

You start by caressing your partner's hair. From there, you work your way to her face, her shoulders, her arms, and her fingers. Then you move to her sides, her lower back, her upper back, and her shoulder blades. Only then do you move down to her buttocks, thus covering all the erogenous zones on the back side of her body. Once you have done that, you move to the front. You don't go right for the nipples, however. They are left to later in the series, teasing your partner's receptivity to greater heights. Do you get the idea?

You start by stroking your partner's hair in order to tune her sensitivity to receive faint signals. Stimulus of the back starts with the lower part of it because of the sacrum, a bone that also acts as a pressure point and that creates and stores a great deal of sexual energy. When you stimulate your partner's feet and legs, you start with her toes, working your way up to her calves and thighs, because you're trying to make her sexual energy flow towards her uterus, heightening her sensitivity.

Erogenous stimulus has meaning and purpose if the order it is performed is true to the female sexual mechanism and psychology. We often get the following question from our male students, however: "What part can I skip if I don't have a lot of time?" This, from students who are trying to learn how to pleasure their partners! All they care about is technique. Men who have never brought a woman to orgasm have in common a fundamental obtuseness regarding strategy. No matter how great your skills are, if you apply them incorrectly, their effectiveness is going to be worse than negligible.

Something men need to know: tactics (techniques) without strategy is pointless.

"Ticklish" is the Gateway to Pleasure

I often get the following from my beginning male students: "Whenever my partner and I engage in foreplay, she tells me it tickles. What am I doing wrong?"

First, I've got to say that there are too many cowards out there who're ready to give up when they don't immediately get the reaction they want. It's beyond naïve to think you can make your partner writhe and moan like a porn star with a little touching and licking. Guys, get real!

To start with, "it tickles" isn't a bad initial reaction at all. It's proof that your stimulus to the skin is being transmitted to the brain properly; it's the stage before "pleasure." When I encounter a woman who reacts that way, I give myself an internal high-five.

There are, of course, some women (not many, thankfully) who are born incapable of feeling sexual arousal—actual, clinical cases of frigidity. Such women don't feel anything when you touch them.

That's why *any* reaction—including "it tickles"—is the gateway to pleasure. It's up to you to stride through the gate and stroll on. Stimulating the feminine body requires all the skills of a top-notch chef preparing a soup: you make fine adjustments to the heat and seasonings; you don't rush to take the pot off the flame before the soup has cooked to perfection. You have to apply the same care to your partner's body so it's "done to perfection."

If your partner tells you it tickles, don't just sit there sucking your thumb. You should be pumping your fist in the air because you've elicited a positive reaction. On the other hand, don't try to explain to her that the ticklish feeling is the first step toward an erogenous reaction. There's no room in bed for theorizing.

In sex just as in love, it's important to know when to back down. Your partner experiences something as ticklish because her brain is unprepared for the power of the signals being received from the site of stimulation. The imbalance arises because she's not yet in an aroused state. The potential for sexual stimulation remains that: potential. In order to put your partner in the mood, you first have to put her in a more relaxed frame of mind.

The technique I recommend is "Palm Touch Stimulation." We've all seen how a crying baby is soothed when its mother gently rubs its back or tummy with the palm of her hand. The principle here is the same. Rubbing your partner's back with the palm of your hand is a very effective way of relaxing her. That doesn't mean you should rub randomly all over the place. There's a technique.

The most fundamental thing is to keep the depression in the palm of your hand pressed tightly against your partner's skin. This is very important. The airtight contact of the entire surface of your palm, combined with a modicum of pressure, is vital. Imagine your palm as a suction cup, and apply stimulation to your partner's back, abdomen, or sides using a lazy clockwise motion in large circles.

More specifically, lie on the bed next to your partner and apply the technique with your arm extended. It's best if she starts facing down, so you can apply the massage to her back. Do her back, her buttocks, and then the backs of her thighs, always using a large, slow circular motion. The relaxing effect can be heightened if you use baby powder. The method is the same when your partner is facing up. Move from her stomach to her sides, her chest, then down to her thighs. Keep the massaging motion slow and steady. Don't let your quickie male instincts get the better of you—avoid the temptation to use your fingers to stimulate her. Keep the palm of your hand tight against her skin. Remember, the whole point of Palm Touch Stimulation is to relax your partner.

Once she is completely relaxed, she ought to start showing a sensual response to the stimulation. This is your chance to convert "ticklish" to "pleasurable" and to segue into the Adam Touch which I describe later. Don't rush. Do the Palm Touch three times, and the Adam Touch once, then the Palm Touch, and so on, repeating this while keeping an eye on your partner's response. By this point, your partner's "potential" sexual response should be an actual one.

The Palm Touch technique is not just for the bed,

either. It can be performed while clothed, and doing it on your partner's back during your daily activities is a good way to accustom her body to your touch. It will make the transition from "relaxed" to "aroused" a lot smoother during sex.

Visual Arousal

Some men—usually those who believe that the man should be active and the woman passive during sex— react negatively towards offers to stimulate them. There is a tendency among such men to resist expressing their pleasure, even going so far as to pretend they aren't feeling anything when they are on the receiving end. Such men seem to think that it's "unmanly" to vocalize their pleasure just because they're feeling good.

It isn't very fair to expect your partner to express her pleasure to you, but not to want to reciprocate in kind. From the point of view of enjoying sex, it's also a waste not to. Women get excited, too, when they see their partners in a state of arousal. Excitement equals the brain becoming more receptive to sexual stimulus, which can only be a good thing, since your partner becomes more sensitive to your touch.

In many cases, men do want their partner to take a more proactive role, but to their disappointment, the partner will not. Let me be very clear: if you give your partner the kind of good sex she really wants, she will reciprocate without your asking.

Humans are at bottom sexual animals. Sometimes we want to do things that would be embarrassing for others to see. We obviously can't do those things in public, so we suppress those urges. One difference between men and women is that women have an easier time suppressing those urges than men. If a man fails to give his partner so much pleasure that her instincts overcome her intellect, she brings that suppressive faculty into bed.

Worse than Sticks and Stones

From the frequency of the complaints I've heard from women, I know how often men hurt women by saying things that are lacking in consideration—to say the least.

"What are you, frigid?"

"There's something wrong with you."

"I did all that, and you *still* can't come?"

These are just some of the printable examples of the horrible things men say to women. As a man, I feel equal doses of shame and anger at this. Let me give you a typical example.

A married couple had been married for twenty years. The husband was fifty-five, and the wife, fifty-two. They

came to me worried that the wife might be frigid. I applied
my massage and not only was she not frigid, she was the
kind of woman no man would ever want to let go! She
was very erotic and climaxed over and over. Her husband
was holding her hand the whole time and was stunned by
the sight of his wife reacting like he'd never seen before.
He had been married to her for twenty years but had
never known about her erogenous zones. I should point
out that these two were having sex more regularly than
other couples their age. Nevertheless, they came to me,
the husband thinking his wife might be frigid, the wife
sharing the same worry. Twenty years! An interesting
side-note: the husband was an ob-gyn.

I've said it before, and I'll say it again: all women's
bodies are designed to feel pleasure. If they don't feel
something, it is due to their partner's ignorance and lack
of sexual technique. Putting aside questions of technique,
no matter how sexually ignorant a man may be, or how
low his skill level, if he is considerate toward his partner,
she will not be dissatisfied with him and he will not hurt
her. It's inexcusable for a man to try to cover up his own
lack of technique and ignorance by directing hurtful words
at his partner.

Women are far more delicate than men may think.
They are more likely to keep their worries and troubles
to themselves, and even throwaway comments by men
can hurt them very much. Such wounds take time to heal,

and until they do, the woman will shut herself off from her partner emotionally and sexually. Naturally, she will henceforth find it harder to respond to sexual stimuli. And that's not all. She's thereby being deprived of the universal right and freedom to *enjoy sex*.

Not much better is the man who persistently interrogates her about whether she enjoyed herself or climaxed. It's undoubtedly an expression of the man's sense of inadequacy, but think of it from her point of view—asked point-blank if you liked the sex, would you answer "no," even if the sex was horrible? You'd say it was great and that of course you climaxed. For the sake of peace on earth, it's high time we moved beyond sex only designed to satisfy men.

And that's exactly what my mission is: to put an end to incompetent sex.

Chapter Three

An Invitation to ſlow ſex

Start by Renouncing Ejaculation

Why do we have sex? Because it feels good, is one obvious answer. But does the typical male of the species actually achieve the pleasure he's looking for through sex? The answer's a lot murkier than you might think.

In the last two chapters I discussed the state of sex today and its attendant misconceptions, the "junk sex" that causes women so much dissatisfaction. What I really want to communicate through this book, however, is that most men who think that sex is pleasurable are actually missing out on the true pleasure that sex can bring. And I have no doubt that many men—even if only subconsciously—want to have better sex. So why can't they? The problem stems from most men's "goal" in having sex. We push the wrong button, and everything goes wrong: our techniques miss their target, and we miss out on the essential pleasures sex can bring.

The biggest misconception brought about by junk sex today is that the primary goal of sex is ejaculation. You might be thinking, "Well, it *is* sex, right? Isn't ejaculating part of that?" Think about it for a second. Male ejaculation is a pretty simple thing compared to the complex, multi-layered climaxes women experience. The real pleasure of sex is in making these two very different gear wheels spin together, but it's also one of the major difficulties sex presents. The two gear wheels aren't turning in unison when not only men but women, too, think that all there is to sex is for the man to ejaculate.

A man's instinctive desire to penetrate his partner as soon as possible, and to ejaculate as soon as possible, inexorably leads to a reduction in the length of time it takes to have sex. For a woman to experience true pleasure, however, this male-centered time allotment is too short. The end result is neglect of women's sexual gratification. To return to the metaphor of the gears, the man's wheel is spinning furiously, while the woman's is untouched and barely turning at all.

As long as men think only of ejaculation as their primary goal, it will be impossible to make the female wheel spin at full speed. It's not just women who suffer, either. Men suffer terribly by missing out on the chance to witness their partners experiencing sensual bliss.

The first thing I tell my male students is to forget about their own ejaculation. When I say this, a sudden quiet usually descends on the room. "What? Don't ejaculate?" They have trouble grasping what's being said. The average reaction is stunned silence, every mouth in the room agape. It's a natural reaction, considering that the students assume ejaculation is an essential component of sex; their reaction demonstrates this. Nevertheless, renouncing ejaculation is the first step in the Slow Sex method for gaining the kind of pleasure and happiness that can't be achieved through ordinary sex.

What is "ideal sex"? Ideal sex is sex that satisfies both the man and the woman—that focuses on each other's pleasures and forgets the clock. Since "forgetting the clock" is an important aspect of enjoying sex, it's important to eliminate the barrier called ejaculation.

Don't get me wrong, though. I'm not saying that ejaculation is bad in and of itself. Nor am I saying you should avoid it at all costs. Demanding that men have sex without ejaculating is cruel (and definitely unusual), but it has the impact needed to cure their mind and body of the poison of junk sex so that they can enjoy real sex. Getting rid of that barrier and letting yourself focus on a world of sensuality with a free mind in the free flow of time is the only way to get you to enjoy sex on a higher plane. In other words, I want you to know that there exists an entire galaxy of pleasure out there whose space can only be reached if you have sex with no thought for your own ejaculation.

The ideal attitude is to think of ejaculation as a bonus. Moreover, if you put the Slow Sex method I describe in this book into practice, the orgasm you will experience will be nothing like any pleasure you have ever known.

Don't Try to Make Her Orgasm

Just like their male partners, women also tend to obsess about orgasm. In life, we have a habit of dividing matters into ones in which the process is more important than the result and ones in which the result is paramount. These days we tend to place sex in the latter category.

Just as an obsessive focus on ejaculation on the man's part makes for boring sex, over-obsessing on orgasm can stop a woman from simply enjoying sex. Let's look at a typical junk sex scenario.

Your partner performs fellatio on you, you return the favor with some cunnilingus, bringing her to orgasm; then you penetrate her and ejaculate. You orgasm, she orgasms—in terms of the kind of sex that predominates today, passing grades all around. But I beg to differ. From my point of view, this is nothing but mutual masturbation. You and your partner both take the goal of sex to be orgasm, and the whole of sex is reduced to a vacuous point. Is this kind of sex really any good? Does it bring anyone pleasure? If it's a one-night stand, you might be able to derive some kind of satisfaction from it, but if you're doing this with a long-term partner, it's only a matter of time before you both get tired of the repetition of the unimaginative refrain.

In the previous chapter I touched on the fact that orgasm and pleasure are different things. A man can easily ejaculate if his penis is stroked vigorously, and a woman can easily orgasm if her clitoris is stimulated by her partner's tongue. That's beginner sex, understandable in a young couple without much experience. Each partner is focused on his or her own pleasure. But mature adults should be aiming for sex that's on a higher plane. You can dramatically improve your sexual technique by focusing on the sensations capable of giving your partner unlimited pleasure, using your knowledge and skills and forgetting about your own ejaculation (a momentary pleasure). Needless to say, women far prefer being with an experienced, mature man to being with a fumbling, unskilled boy, and your reputation will reflect this.

Men, too, can obsess about making their partners orgasm. There's nothing wrong with wanting to give your partner this pleasure, of course, but if the desire is not accompanied by the requisite skills and know-how regarding the female sexual mechanism, it can be a problem. As I said, men who labor under the misconception that "the stronger the stimulus, the greater the pleasure" tend to stimulate the clitoris or vagina aggressively; this not only does *not* feel good, it can actually cause pain. There might be women out there who like that kind of thing and who can reach orgasm from stimulus that borders on violence. Men should know, however, that the level of pleasure they generally give their partners through their incorrect techniques is not that different from the pleasure women can give themselves through masturbating.

In the course of my work I listen to a lot of women, and naturally I'm amazed by the number of women who confide to me that masturbating feels better than sex with their partner (although they could never tell him that). Once they have experienced my orgasm technique, these women realize the mistake of comparing sex and masturbation, but it's not surprising that they consider themselves more technically skilled than their partners. The only kind of sex they know is junk sex.

After hearing this explanation, men (logically) ask, "So how do you give a woman a high-level orgasm?" and I answer, "By not trying to give her an orgasm." I'm not playing the Zen master when I say that, though. Here's something I've often heard women tell each other, but which rarely reaches men's ears: "I know he's really trying hard to make me orgasm, but when I see that desperate look in his eyes, it kind of freaks me out."

It's worth restating: women's bodies and minds are very delicate. Trying to force a woman to reach orgasm is only going to be a burden on her and make her less receptive. Change your approach from "I'm going to make you come no matter what!" to "I'm going to make you feel good for a long time," and you'll be able to impart stimulus that matches her sexual mechanism more closely.

I describe specific techniques later on, but this change in your awareness alone will suffice to raise your sexual skill level.

The Problem with "Fore"-Play

One of the important resolutions of Slow Sex is to forget the clock and enjoy sex. It takes time to get your partner's gear wheel turning. Letting your partner know that she has all the time in the world has a psychologically relaxing effect and puts her in a state of mind that more efficiently converts stimulus into sexual pleasure.

Accordingly, I want to shed a spotlight on what's commonly known as "foreplay" today. For better or for worse, people tend to take things literally. In the case of "foreplay," most men have subconsciously assumed that foreplay is what you do *before* engaging in penetrative sex. This cements the notion that the "correct" order of the different stages of a sexual encounter is: foreplay, penetration, ejaculation. The reason there are so many men for whom foreplay is reduced almost to a formality

preceding penetration—despite sincerely wanting to give
their partner an orgasm—is that this preconception of
foreplay has taken the fun and freedom out of sex. This
may sound harsh, but there's not much difference between
the man who spends five minutes on foreplay and the man
who spends thirty-five minutes on it, since both view it as
nothing more than something you do before penetrating
your partner.

The Slow Sex I propose is sex for the sake of *enjoying
sex*. This means sex where both partners experience
pleasure without making ejaculation a goal. Put simply,
it's sex that is one long session of foreplay. In ideal sex, you
and your partner are mutually aroused through mutual
stimulation. The word "foreplay" is totally inappropriate
if we want to eliminate time limits and preconceptions
about the order various acts should be performed in. That's
why I have created the word "loveplay" as a substitute.
This turns the concept on its head by getting rid of all the
artificial notions—"before vs. after penetration," "during
penetration," and so on—and places this "loveplay,"
during which you and your partner spend as much time
as possible stimulating each other's bodies, at the heart of
sex.

Slow Sex is sex in which loveplay goes on and on. The
essence of sex is forgetting the clock and enjoying this non-
stop loveplay. This might be hard for someone used to junk
sex to understand, but once you grasp this fundamental

principle, you'll be able to reconceptualize penetration as "vaginal stimulation using the penis." That's the key to converting penetration, which is currently nothing more really than using your partner's vagina to masturbate, into real sex, in which both you and your partner share pleasure.

Sex is the Interaction of Sexual Energy

Now we're getting to the core of what sex is all about. This is the most important part in the book, so read carefully. There's a reason I haven't touched on this until now: namely, it's impossible to understand what I'm about to discuss if you think junk sex is the way sex is supposed to be. If you've read this far, however, you've been at least partially liberated from the poisonous effects of junk sex.

That's the assumption I'm making going into the following discussion.

Sex is not the simple friction of skin against skin, as typified by thrusting the penis into the vagina. The real pleasure of sex comes from causing the positive and negative sexual energies you and your partner have from birth to circulate through your bodies.

All right, so maybe this talk of "sexual energy" has left you with a furrowed brow. But the truth is that your pleasure deepens proportionately to the total increase in sexual energy you and your partner produce.

This energy isn't some sparkly aura floating in the air, so it might be hard to get a handle on what I mean by it. Let's start by defining this energy as something that is produced by your feelings and emotions. Remember high school, when just thinking about that girl in chemistry class set your heart racing? That is the energy I'm talking about. Remember the almost electrical surge that shot through you when you held her hand for the first time? That's what I'm talking about.

When you're in a relationship with a woman and the sex is great, you might opine that your bodies are a perfect match. If you don't know about sexual energy, then that's a natural way to express the feeling, but the fact of the matter is that it doesn't have anything to do with your body. Your respective energies are on complementary wavelengths and are interacting, without your even being aware of it, and the result is good sex—and not just sex, either. In your work and social relationships, this energy plays a major role. Have you ever noticed how you immediately get along with some people, when with others you know right away that you'll never get along? That's the same effect.

Let's look at a more specific case. When you first have sex with a woman, be it someone you've longed after for years or someone you just picked up at a bar that night, the sex is usually great, isn't it? That's because you are both in a heightened emotional state and your sexual energies are naturally amplified. You've probably noticed how the second and third times aren't as great, especially because the first time was mind-blowing. Your level of excitement has dropped off compared to the first time, and your level of sexual energy has returned to normal.

I keep repeating that the first step to Slow Sex is forgetting the clock because the more time you spend on sexual pleasure, the greater your sexual energy will be. For a woman's body, greater sexual energy equals greater sensitivity and receptiveness. A "virtuous circle" emerges in direct contrast to the "vicious circle" created by junk sex, which is an accumulation of dissatisfaction and stress.

You probably didn't know this, and it's likely that nobody ever told you, but it's no exaggeration to say that how great the sex is depends on how high you can raise your and your partner's sexual energy levels through loveplay. You might not be able to see it with your eyes, but it's a law that no one can break. The most hallowed, esoteric technique in Slow Sex is the ability to control this invisible sexual energy at will.

You might think all this talk of "energy" sounds a bit fishy. I used to be the same way until something happened that proved that it exists.

This is actually kind of embarrassing, but I'll tell you the story to better enable you to understand the existence of this energy. It happened when I was still in my twenties. Although no one will believe me now, I suffered from freakishly premature ejaculation. I couldn't even last a minute. I was already married at that time, and sex with my wife always ended with an awkward smile from her. I had tried all sorts of things to overcome this shortcoming, but nothing worked, and I had almost given up. No, I had given up completely. It was around then that I met a particular woman. One thing led to another, and—miracle of miracles—when I had sex with her, I was able to hold out as long as I wanted. Our encounter wasn't just a "fling," either. She was a very passionate woman, and the sex was bolder and more intense than anything I had ever experienced, which was reflected in my level of arousal. And my penis, which ordinarily would release its load upon penetration, held out for longer than I thought possible. I felt that something inside me had changed, that my sexual constitution had undergone a transformation for the better.

The next day, I had sex with my wife, wanting to test this feeling against reality, and the result was…the same as always. What had happened? I began giving the problem serious thought, and I noticed one difference in particular: the length of our kisses. My wife wasn't particularly fond of kissing, so we almost never kissed during sex. In contrast, the woman I was having the affair with loved kissing and wanted me to kiss her even while I was penetrating her. I thought about other differences. When I had sex with my wife, I felt a kind of heat concentrated in my lower abdomen that caused me to ejaculate very quickly. With the other woman, I felt the heat equally distributed over my entire body. That's when I realized that it's something other than crude friction that is related to ejaculatory endurance, and that the something is "energy." I hypothesized that the energy that accumulated in my lower abdomen interacted with that of my new partner through extended periods of kissing and that the interaction caused it to flow throughout our bodies.

Thereafter—with the consent of my very understanding wife—I tested out my hypothesis with many women, and I successfully proved that my hypothesis was correct. That was the starting point of who I am now.

I'm the first to admit that talking about "energies" flowing through your body inspires the kind of suspicion that stories about ghosts and supernatural powers do. I use the term "sexual energy," which has a bit more of a scientific ring than, say, *ki*, but even then, most people have to experience it to believe it. That doesn't mean it doesn't exist. *Ki* does exist, and everyone produces it.

So, even if you're not fully convinced, at least give me the benefit of the doubt. An awareness of *ki* will take your sexual pleasure to a level you've never experienced before. If you are aware that the contact of your penis with your partner's vagina is not mere friction but is actually the site of interaction of your and your partner's *ki*, your sex life will change completely.

Developing the Erogenous Brain

By now you are at least vaguely aware of the dramatic effect sexual energy (*ki*) has on sex. In this section, I will go into further detail about the relationship between sexual energy and the female sexual mechanism.

Let's recall: a woman doesn't feel pleasure at her erogenous zones, but rather in her brain. Feelings of pleasure don't exist on the skin. They exist in the brain. In this book, I call this nerve center of pleasure in the brain, where stimulation is recognized as pleasure, the "erogenous brain." People talk about women being more, or less, sensitive to stimulus. Aside from being an incorrect description of the female sexual mechanism, this way of thinking is the source of many other misconceptions. Experiencing pleasure, not feeling anything, even feeling ticklish—these are all judgments made in the brain. I want you to remember this.

There is no such thing as a woman with a very sensitive clitoris, or nipples that are not sensitive. Whether or not something feels good, and the degree to which it does, depend on whether or not a person's "erogenous brain" has developed far enough to experience stimulation received by the erogenous zones as pleasurable. All women's bodies are designed so that their erogenous zones can transmit pleasure during sex once they are fully mature.

So why are some women more sensitive than others? It

depends on the extent of their sexual experience, how early they began showing an interest in the opposite sex, when they started masturbating, whether they were surrounded by many members of the opposite sex while growing up, and many other factors that affect the maturity of their erogenous brain. That's why some women love sex right from their first experience, while others hate it even after having sex with dozens of men.

In other words, sensitivity is a question of how developed a woman's erogenous brain is. No matter how quiet, shy, or intellectual a woman may ordinarily be, if you succeed in fully developing her erogenous brain, she will turn into an erotic animal in bed.

So how is this done? The most effective method is to provide scrupulous stimulation to each of the numerous erogenous zones scattered all over her body. For example, if she gets pleasure from stimulus to her nipples, that means that the "circuit" between her nipples and her erogenous brain has been opened up. The many erogenous zones all over her body are interconnected. When they are successfully linked up, the entire surface of her body will be a network of erogenous zones. I call this opening up the erogenous routes. The more these routes between the erogenous zones and the erogenous brain are opened up, the greater the functionality of the erogenous brain. In other words, not only will the woman start feeling erogenous pleasure all over her body, but the intensity of the sensation will increase.

"Providing scrupulous stimulation to each of the numerous erogenous zones" may sound like a mind-numbingly time-consuming process, but that's not the case. As little as thirty minutes of loveplay can suffice. It's just that foreplay in its current form, which barely lasts fifteen minutes on average and focuses too much on the breasts and clitoris, does not include any of the things I discuss. Think about your pattern—how many parts of her body have you never even once touched? You could put it down to your preferences, but if your loveplay includes only those places you want to touch, or where you get a good reaction, you'll never be able to develop your partner's erogenous routes. And this is why there are so many women who are perfectly healthy in all respects who still think they're frigid.

All men love women who are sensitive to sexual stimulus, which is why I'm surprised that no one has ever tried to spread the knowledge and techniques needed to make women more sensitive. I will describe two techniques for making your partner's body one uninterrupted erogenous zone.

I call the first one the "Simultaneous Method" because it involves stimulating two places at once: one zone where your partner already feels pleasure, and another zone that hasn't been developed yet. Areas that produce pleasure are already joined to the erogenous brain through the nerves, while areas that don't produce pleasure are that way because their erogenous routes are cut off. By stimulating one of each simultaneously, it's possible to connect the two zones and create an erogenous route between them.

The second technique is the "Surround and Conquer Method" and involves gradually broadening the area of stimulation of an erogenous zone to include other zones that don't produce pleasure. For example, if your partner feels pleasure from stimulation of her nipples, but is ticklish on her sides, you would gradually expand the scope of stimulation from the nipple to the side. The principle is the same as the Simultaneous Method in that areas that previously didn't produce pleasure begin to do so.

In Chapter Four I describe the Adam Touch, a hand technique I designed in order to develop the erogenous brain, and I hope you can put it to use in helping your partner get the most out of her erogenous brain.

Sex as Relaxation

We live in an age of relaxation. From puppies to bath oils to big-screen TVs, people are looking for ways to de-stress and relax. In this regard, nothing beats sex. It is the original relaxation method, but you would never guess that from the way people have sex today—it's become a major source of stress! There are many women who would prefer to fall asleep in their partner's arms than have sex as a means of comfort. It's sad but true.

Say the word "relaxation," and most people think of hot baths and poolside naps, but sex actually has a more relaxing effect than any of that. The secret: the *ki* energy I discussed above. Yoga is one familiar example of using energy to relax, but in yoga you meditate in order to control the flow of energy through your body. Taichi operates on the same principle. Yoga and Taichi are well-known ways to maintain your health, but with sex you don't have to learn their complicated methods to get your energy flowing. Plus, you're using your partner's energy, too. As a result, your tense, fatigued autonomous nervous system unwinds, and hormone secretion is promoted. It feels good and *is* good for you. Slow Sex makes your energy flow for a long period of time, naturally warming up your body. You feel the warmth down to the tips of your toes. By keeping warm in this way, you improve your health and maintain your beauty in addition to gaining a deep sense of satisfaction and contentment. In this sense, Slow Sex is far better than any bath or pool.

Junk sex infects our culture like a virus. The man pumps away aggressively at his partner, drenching himself in sweat—sweat from simple exertion and not from the power of his *ki* energy. The woman, on the other hand, doesn't sweat at all, so she doesn't even get the release of physical exertion. When I have sex, my partner and I are both equally drenched in sweat.

When you're healthy, you eat well, you sleep well, and you feel refreshed every morning. Your sex drive is also a barometer of your health. These days, however, more and more couples aren't having sex at all even though they're in the prime of youth. They've simply given up on it—not a good thing. No longer caring about sex has a drastic effect on hormone secretion in both men and women, causing the body to age quicker. As an anti-aging method (which admittedly is another recent fad), few things are better than Slow Sex.

Human Sex and Animal Sex

Like other animals, humans mate in order to reproduce, but only humans have sex for fun. Other ani-mals obey their instincts and find a partner for repro-duction during mating season and the act itself is over almost as soon as it starts. Humans, on the other hand, seek pleasure and love in sex, sharing happiness with their partners. The differences between human sex and animal sex are therefore profound.

I'm not saying this because I think humans are somehow better than other animals. However, only humans can discover the dignity of life through our ability to enjoy sex. By not enjoying sex properly, we're losing some of that human dignity, as can be seen in the phenomenon of junk sex. Putting our own pleasure before all else, and engaging in sex that is focused only on our own ejaculation without a thought for our partners, cannot be in any way called dignified.

By maintaining the proper view of sex and being very observant about the sexual and physiological differences between ourselves and our partners, we will not only discover the charm and beauty of the female body, but also be rewarded with a sense of being alive in the moment. There's no reason to complicate sex, but it's not as simple as you think, either.

Sex is the Greatest Gift from God

Whenever I perform an orgasm massage on a woman, I wonder why women are so much more sensitive to sexual stimulus than men.

Men have a single erogenous center, while women's erogenous zones are spread all over their bodies, from their hair to their toes—all of it one uninterrupted erogenous zone. Not only that, but women can achieve pleasure on an incomparably higher plane than men. They writhe, they tremble, they moan with a rapturous look on their face... Every time I witness a sensuality beyond men's understanding, I wish I could experience it, too.

If the only purpose of sex were to reproduce, then there wouldn't be a need for women to be so sensitive to stimulus. Why is it so? I think God designed the female body for it to be loved by men. That's the only way I can explain to myself why there are so many erogenous zones all over the female body, why the pleasure derived from each one is unique, and why there are very powerful erogenous zones in places which can only be reached by a finger or a penis.

The more I explore the mysteries of the female body, the more convinced I become that sex is the greatest gift God has given to us humans. Sex is the ultimate creative expression, a dance that joins body and mind.

The world is full of diversions. If you have the money, you can do almost anything. You can walk into town and eat food from around the world and visit places of amusement. You can travel to distant lands. But does any of this bring us true happiness?

Just the other day I watched a TV show about a housewife who was addicted to an online social networking site. She just sat in front of the computer, ignoring her kids even if they needed something. That's right! She chose a faceless, nameless somebody on the internet over her own children! Am I the only one who is shocked by such warped family relations? But that woman is not unique. Everybody wants to be loved and to feel a connection with others, but communicating with members of the opposite sex can be difficult. You have relationship troubles, you give up, you're afraid of getting hurt, so you satisfy your inner urges in a virtual world. It's a vicious circle that is threatening to control our lives.

I'll say it again. Sex is the greatest gift God has given us. You need neither status nor fame nor money to enjoy sex. All you have to do is want it. If you not only want to be loved but have an active desire to love the woman you are with, then sex can bring you not only pleasure, but happiness as well.

How many people in the world truly feel happy? The majority might not even know what it is to be happy—scary, but entirely possible. That's why I want all men and women to know that there is a place you can find true happiness and that it's within everyone's reach.

Controlling Your Ejaculation

No matter how much you know about sex or how good you are at enjoying it, if you suffer from premature ejaculation, you'll miss out on the best part of Slow Sex.

Some men try to stave off the inevitable by thrusting their hips slowly, almost hesitantly. But even if that worked, it wouldn't be the same as the "extended intercourse" made possible by Slow Sex, in which you spend a long time with your partner enjoying the feel of your penis in her vagina.

Learning how to control your ejaculation is your duty as a man and a requisite for good sex.

Naturally, there's no man alive who doesn't wish to hold out longer, but that doesn't stop quite a few men from giving up. As I confessed above, I used to suffer from almost incapacitating premature ejaculation (less than a minute). My self-esteem and self-confidence were in tatters and I had almost given up hope. Today, I have gained so much control that I can engage in intercourse for two, even three hours at a time.

Through a lot of trial and error, I developed two training methods for overcoming premature ejaculation. They can be performed alone.

The autonomous nervous system that controls the state of your body can be controlled through breathing. Mastering a breathing technique that includes elements of tantric yoga will help you bring your parasympathetic nervous system to the fore, making it possible to suppress arousal. This breathing method is absolutely necessary when controlling ejaculation.

The way it is done is very simple.

A. Breathing Technique for Overcoming Premature Ejaculation
1. Inhale, imagining that your lungs are in your head and that you are sucking the air in through your anus and up through your backbone to your head.

2. Exhale slowly, counting to seven.

3. Constrict your anus ten times rhythmically.

4. Repeat this whenever you feel yourself about to ejaculate.

That's all there is to it. Breathing in is the hardest part, but you'll get the hang of it after a few tries. When you breathe in, your sympathetic nervous system comes to the fore, and when you breathe out, your parasympathetic nervous system comes to the fore. Accordingly, it's important to inhale quickly, and let the air out as slowly as possible.

B. Penis Stiffness Training

1. Put massage oil on the palm of your hand and your penis and stimulate yourself, focusing on the head of your penis.

2. When you feel yourself about to ejaculate, stop your hand and repeat Method A above.

3. Do this for at least 15 minutes.

4. Once you are accustomed to it, end the training without ejaculating.

These two training methods will build the resistance of your penis to stimulus and give you greater endurance to control your ejaculation. Use these methods when you masturbate. I guarantee you will see results, and I should know, because I had badly premature ejaculation. That said, premature ejaculation is not such a simple problem that you will overcome it right away. For some people, it takes two weeks. In other cases, people only see results after six months of continuous training. The important thing is not to give up.

You can do this training by yourself, but my advice is to get help from your partner. Premature ejaculation can give a man a serious complex. It's understandable if you don't want anyone to know about your complex, especially women. Still, no matter how good your excuses, every time you have sex, your partner will know. It's a safe bet that your partner is just pretending not to notice, in order not to hurt you. So instead of keeping it to yourself and letting it fester, just come out into the open and admit your problem. There is no way sex will ever be pleasurable if it's accompanied by a complex about premature ejaculation and the resultant pressure. Come clean with your partner, and eliminate that pressure. Then you can focus all your energy and attention on facing the complex—namely, by getting help from your partner when conducting the penis stiffness training above. Getting rid of taboos between you and your partner will have the added benefit of increasing your love.

Coming clean to your partner may be embarrassing for a minute, but not conquering your premature ejaculation will embarrass you every time you have sex.

True Sex Will Drive Them Wild

Have you ever made a woman scream from pleasure? I don't mean this metaphorically—not "Mmm, that's good!" or "Oh yeah, I'm coming!" I mean a primal, animal scream. Not many men have. And not many women have ever experienced the kind of orgasm that would cause them to scream like that.

Let me tell you something.

In a previous chapter I said that 95% of women who think they might be frigid are perfectly fine. In other words, most women have ordinary sensitivity to sexual stimulus. The problem is that both men and women underestimate what "ordinary" means. Most women have the potential to experience scream-inducing orgasms. If a woman screams during orgasm, men tend to be amazed by how open she is, but screaming is not that amazing. In fact, screaming is a phenomenon that any woman can attain if her erogenous brain is developed and her erogenous routes are all opened up. If a woman is filled up with sexual energy, she will naturally let out a wild scream, just as a cup overflows with water when filled to the top.

Rather than being surprised, men should be ashamed that they have never heard a woman scream this way, since it isn't difficult to bring about. The only kind of stimulation women usually receive is the rough bumbling of their partners trying to make them reach orgasm as quickly as possible, so men unsurprisingly never get the chance to hear their partner's true voice.

Let's review. Your ability to make a woman feel pleasure, to give her great sex, depends on your ability to amplify her sexual energy. This is done by supplying her with faint, exquisite physical stimulus. Sexual energy is transmitted from your fingers to each of her erogenous zones. Put simply, quit trying to make your partner orgasm, and focus on giving her pleasure. This new type of loveplay will open up her erogenous brain and fill her body with sexual energy. When her body is brimming with sexual energy, she will effortlessly achieve an explosive orgasm.

I can't even count the number of times I've heard women scream so raucously during orgasm that I thought the walls were going to come down. They try to cover their mouths, but that doesn't work, so I give them a towel to scream into. That doesn't work either. Scream after scream issues forth from their mouths, oblivious to our efforts to muffle them. The point of this story is that these women who scream so much that they come to fear that the neighbors might complain were all once students in our "frigidity therapy" class. Young professional women who have never once felt pleasure during sex, despite having had encounters with many men; wives married for decades who have never experienced an orgasm; women who have never felt anything despite the strenuous efforts of their boyfriends or husbands: they all begin screaming with pleasure as soon as I service them.

That's the power of proper technique.

Don't misunderstand, though. I'm not saying that my technique cures women of their frigidity so that they can finally have such orgasms. The women were not frigid to begin with. They were normal in every respect. All I did was release the potential they already had that their partners' technique could not bring out.

Women are blessed with countless erogenous zones. A woman's entire body is one continuous erogenous zone. Most men are vaguely aware of this, but they make the mistake of thinking that they can touch a woman just anywhere. The words "countless" and "entire body" are deceptively simple. The result is that men don't think before they touch. The erogenous zones may be "countless" in number, but each one is a small, well-defined zone. You can't provide pinpoint stimulus if you're sloppy. You might retort that if a woman's entire body is an erogenous zone, all you need to do is provide stimulus over her entire body and you'll hit the right place. Let's be accurate about this. You might hit the right spot, but it will only be for an instant, and that's not enough. You have to focus your energies on that one spot in order to develop your partner's erogenous brain and open up her erogenous routes.

It's vital that you focus all your attention on finding those small erogenous zones by fine-tuning your loveplay and keeping a close eye (and ear) on your partner's response. That's the biggest difference between someone capable of making any woman scream with pleasure (i.e., me) and most men, who have never once succeeded in doing so.

Another story.

Before students at my school practice their loveplay technique on one of the female models we have, we give them technical instruction using mock-ups of the female genitalia. After all, if they don't know what the clitoris, urethra, labia minora, labia majora, and other parts are and where they are located, no amount of practice will help. What's surprising is the number of men who don't know the names and locations of these parts. There are even married men who can't tell you where the clitoris is— the clitoris! When I ask them why, their answer is simple: they've never seen a woman's genitalia in the light.

Makes sense. Most women want the lights off when they have sex. They're probably afraid they'll look fat, or perhaps there are places that they don't want to show to the man they love. So they turn off the lights and crawl under the sheets. That's why there are so many men who have never had the chance to actually see a woman's genitalia in the flesh.

So they fumble around with their hands, and the result is that they have only a vague notion of where things are— forget trying to fine-tune your loveplay while keeping an

eye on your partner's response. To be honest, I pity men
who have to work in the face of such adversity. The fact
remains, however, that unless they do something about it
and start examining all those individual erogenous zones,
their future sex life will remain as dark as the rooms they
have sex in.

If your wife or girlfriend is shy about having the lights
on, then your job is to communicate to her the importance
of being able to see her expression and body.

Screaming isn't just for Women Anymore

We've spoken about women screaming. Now let's talk
about men screaming. It isn't a privilege reserved just
for women. Indeed, men have the same hidden potential
as women do in this area. Granted, the most common
reaction when I tell men that they can scream too is
something along the lines of "yeah, right." Most men don't
realize that men can experience the kind of pleasure that
would make them scream, since all that they have to go on
is the slight grunt of release they know from ejaculating
during sex or masturbation.

I've already explained the relationship to sexual
energy, but all of that applies equally to men. Once sexual
energy is amplified, men can also experience the moaning
kind of orgasm women have.

Let me give you a concrete example. You undoubtedly know from your own experience that the level of pleasure afforded by an orgasm varies depending on who you're having sex with, the situation, and even how you're feeling that day. Some ejaculations leave you with a neat sense of release, while others are more satisfying, and still others might leave you with a feeling of emptiness. All of these things depend on your level of sexual energy.

The sexual energy I have been talking about isn't something that your body produces only when you perform sex "correctly." Your body is producing it all the time—even now. However, since you aren't having sex the right way, your sexual energy is significantly smaller than the energy produced by Slow Sex, making it difficult for you to be aware of that energy.

Even among men who are not aware of their sexual energy, there are minor differences arising from what kind of sex they are having. This can be seen in the varying levels of pleasure they derive from their orgasms.

If you have fully understood sexual energy and the mechanism of pleasure and are already at it, then I can make a guess: the ejaculations you experience are far better than anything you've experienced before, since you are accumulating sexual energy in your body right up to ejaculation. This is more than male ejaculation—it is male orgasm.

Naturally, men will never be able to experience the

devastating pleasure that women feel during orgasm, which is hundreds of times more intense. I can only imagine what it must be like. I'm envious.

Here's something else men might find difficult to imagine: it actually becomes more difficult for women to reach orgasm as the sexual energy building up in their body peaks through Slow Sex, which is for enjoying the pleasure itself. That doesn't mean they aren't feeling good, of course; they are already in a pleasure zone on a much higher plane than the orgasms they experience from junk sex or masturbation. I call this state "being in heaven," and some women stay "in heaven" as long as the loveplay continues. It's a transcendental experience.

There is no doubt that you, too, can experience much better ejaculation than in the past if you use the correct sex techniques, even if the exalted level of women's pleasure will always be out of reach. I sometimes experience thirty seconds or more of bliss after ejaculation. And during those thirty seconds, I'm in there with my partner, screaming my head off.

So how can you achieve this kind of transcendental ejaculation? You have to have the kind of sex where you are stimulating your partner, but where your partner is stimulating you, too. To produce more sexual energy, you and your partner have to work together, passing that energy back and forth. You make that amplified sexual energy circulate between your bodies without letting it accumulate in either body alone.

When a man learns the happiness of focusing his energy on pleasing his partner, watching her beautiful arousal arouses him in turn, creating a great deal of sexual energy. It passes into your partner through your fingers or your penis and is amplified, combining with the sexual energy in your partner's body, where it circulates too. The combined energy is then fed back into you.

Freeing yourself of stereotypical notions like "the man making the woman come" and "men are active, women are passive" and engaging in the two-way interaction of pleasure I describe will enable you to create a flow of pure sexual energy that will be amplified many times over.

Use the proper techniques, and experience this mind-blowing pleasure. You'll never think of ejaculation the same way again.

The Ecstasy of the Aroused Woman

At the beginning of this chapter I told you to renounce ejaculation. For men whose sole purpose in sex is to ejaculate, it might be difficult to imagine that anything could feel better than ejaculating. This, however, is just proof that you have been infected by the ills of junk sex.

What could be better than ejaculation? The answer is simple: watching a woman in a state of extreme arousal.

You might reply that you do that all the time. Perhaps, but now that you know about the erogenous brain and erogenous routes, and the relationship between them and sexual energy, you might be starting to have some doubts about the level of pleasure you are giving your partner.

I just talked about female screaming. One of the things that men worry about is women faking it—either pretending it feels good, or pretending to orgasm. Doubts feed on themselves: "She looks like she's enjoying it, but is she really?" "I asked her if she came, and she said yes, but did she really?" Well, if a woman is screaming in ecstasy, you can be sure she isn't faking it. When a woman's erogenous brain is fully lit up, it's as though her rational faculties fly out the window. Providing accurate and appropriate stimulus of erogenous zones does away with any upper limit on the pleasure a woman can feel. Your partner will become completely receptive, giving herself over to the waves of pleasure washing over her. She simply won't be able to control her reactions, and she certainly won't be able to consciously limit herself to "ladylike" moaning. She has no choice but to reveal the primal, pleasure-craving side of herself that's inscribed in her DNA.

I can say without fear of rebuttal that any man who thinks ejaculation is the pinnacle of sex has never witnessed a woman writhing in the throes of passion as I have described, because if he has—even once—he would know. Just as women cannot inhibit themselves when their arousal mechanism has been turned on through the application of proper technique, men also have it written in their DNA to give a woman more pleasure when they see her truly aroused, with no thought for their own ejaculation.

Sexual Technique and Sex Appeal

I'm a man, and I know that men are a lot more delicate than most women think. When a lack of confidence in your own sexual technique and a strong desire to give your partner pleasure come together, they can create a very serious complex.

At my school we have many students who lack confidence in their sexual technique, and I always marvel at how their demeanor changes once they have learned proper technique. They are like different men. It's not only their demeanor that changes, either. After completing the classes, a good number who had been in no real relationships until then—in some cases virgins well into their thirties—email me telling me that they'd found girlfriends.

It's impossible to overstate the importance of self-confidence in men. It is directly linked to their appeal in the eyes of the opposite sex. That doesn't mean that self-confidence works the same way for all men. Individual values play a large part, but in general, men derive their self-confidence from being rich, good-looking, athletic, famous, powerful, and the like. However, after seeing so many students who have learned the right techniques and how they begin to glow with self-confidence, I'm convinced that there's no single type of self-confidence that can change a man as much as confidence in his sexual technique.

Among my students are men who have the kind of wealth and status that would make other men drool. Still, no matter how haughty they may be before their subordinates at work, or how much wealth they have accumulated, they cannot escape the complexes they have about sexual technique. It's true that in some cases it is exactly those complexes that drive them to become so successful, but that's only in the eyes of others. Inside, the suffering doesn't abate. There's nothing quite as wretched as being a big man whose dizzying social status is totally deflated by abysmal performance in bed.

The book you are holding in your hands right now is a fantastic stroke of luck. Once you have gained a correct understanding of sex and learned proper technique, you will be an unrivaled lover. The self-confidence will change your life.

Chapter Four
The Adam Sex Theory

Arousal and Sensuality Begin with Relaxing

Women's bodies are designed to become more sensitive the more they are aroused. Being aroused means your partner's "erogenous brain" is better able to interpret as sexual stimulation the touch of your fingers and tongue on her skin, which is an erogenous zone. The result is a palpable and very sensitized reaction. I don't think I need to add any more commentary on the truth of this fact.

As a man, you probably already know this. But when it comes down to specific expertise and psychological techniques for bringing a woman to a state of arousal, too often most men are ignorant and unprepared, sometimes just plain dumb.

One typical example of a just plain dumb approach is thinking you can get your partner aroused by showing her pornographic videos. There are so many things wrong with this approach that I don't have the space to describe them all. The idea that you can turn a woman on by having her watch porn is simplistic, to say the least. Thinking that what turns you on will also turn your partner on is self-centered. To begin with, it's fairly common knowledge that more women are turned off by porn than turned on by it, so the approach is likely to have an effect that is the exact opposite of what you intend. Even if we assume for the sake of argument that your partner is actually aroused by watching pornography, what guarantee is there that she will be willing to come out to you about something that she probably thinks of as her "dirty little secret"? The answer, obviously, is "none." The likeliest scenario is that no matter what a woman thinks about porn—whether she loves it or loathes it—her first reaction will be to become tense and feel awkward the minute you press the play button. Men's magazines are full of articles describing the great sex the writer had after he showed his girlfriend a porno movie. These are rare cases. No more than one or two in a hundred will have such experiences. I'll let you in on a little secret if you happened not to know: for the most part, those articles are nothing but pure fantasy on the part of the writer. The "porn strategy" (if you can call it a strategy) only works when a) your partner is interested in pornography and b) you've been divulged this in a prior conversation. Know that if you allow yourself to be fooled by irresponsible media, you're going to pay for it.

What exactly am I branding as ignorant here? In this case, it means not being abreast of the fundamental truth that for a woman to become aroused, there has to be a preceding stage of relaxation—opening up to the partner she's considering having sex with. Relaxation is what makes it possible for her erogenous brain to initiate the preparations for putting her body into a more sensitized state. Only once these preparations are complete is it possible to move to the next step, namely, arousal.

This is what most differentiates women from us men, who are aroused by the mere sight of a woman's cleavage or a simple touch—in other words, who are easily excited by visual and tactile information sent to our brain. Most of the factors contributing to men's ignorance originate in the fact that men assume women are just like themselves when in fact they are radically different creatures.

The reason most guys who go on dates with the intention of "going all the way" fail to reach their goal is that they ignore what I consider to be this fundamental fact: the prologue to sex for women is relaxation. If there's a guy you know who always seems to get the ladies despite not being particularly handsome or cool, observe what he says and does. You'll probably notice that even though he jokes around with a woman, he's always considerate, he listens patiently to what she has to say, and so on. In other words, he's deploying techniques for putting the woman at ease and helping her relax, even if he's doing it unconsciously.

Incidentally, many of the women who come to my school suffer from "frigidity," and what I struggle with most when helping them out is not what sexual techniques to use on them, but how to help them de-stress and get them to relax. A woman's most faithful companions during sex are her insecurities—about reaching orgasm, about what her partner thinks of her, about her own body, about potential pain, about past bad experiences, etc. The list is endless. It is vital for a woman to be able to sweep all that tension aside if she is to enjoy sex that is unrestrained and liberating.

It's important for you to be conscious that the natural pull of love brings two people together on the basis of feelings of mutual trust, consideration, comfort, and being at ease together. Take a hard look at the incorrect techniques you have used in the past to arouse your partners as quickly as possible. If you are currently in a relationship, try talking about methods that might help both of you to relax. This in itself can be pleasurable and can help to create bridges of sexual communication that are sorely lacking today.

Your Fingers for Loveplay, Your Mouth for Expressions of Love

When you have sex, do you use your fingers or mouth (tongue) more? If you're like most men, you probably use your mouth more often. It could be called almost an animal instinct for a man to lick a nipple when he sees one. Considering the spectrum of sex manuals on the market today teaching oral technique, it's inevitable that men are so fond of oral sex. Nevertheless, the number-one guaranteed method to give a woman pleasure is to apply just the right amount of continuous stimulation to a very specific location. It goes without saying that your fingers are better suited to this than your mouth. When it comes to dexterity, few tools beat the human finger, which is equipped with motor skills so fine it can be used to write on grains of rice. There is also the "sexual energy" that stimulates a woman's erogenous brain, and although not visible, fingers exude it in much larger quantities than the tongue. The conclusion is that in terms of agility and production of sexual energy, your fingers are best suited to caressing your partner's erogenous zones.

If definitive textbooks on sex existed, the rules they'd expound on the very first page would be the ones that are unknown to most men.

Just so I'm not misunderstood, let me state that I'm not saying oral sex is bad. Fellatio and cunnilingus are great techniques that involve physical stimulation as well factors of visual stimulation, and both demand skilled use of the tongue. The mouth, in fact, is an ideal organ for expressing your love. However, your tongue is a lot rougher than you might imagine, and stimulus provided with it lacks precision and pacing. It also has another fatal drawback. When performing oral sex, your face is too close to your partner's body for you to see how she is reacting. Using your fingers allows you a much broader visual field for observing your partner's reactions. Your fingers, many times more agile than your tongue, makes them ideal for developing and opening up your partner's erogenous routes.

At my school, we teach our students on the first day that "your fingers are for loveplay, and your mouth is for expressions of love." The ideal is to understand the strengths and advantages of your fingers and tongue and to use them together in the best way possible.

In the next section, we will take a close look at the "Adam Touch," the ultimate hand technique.

The Adam Touch—Making It Possible for Women to Reach Orgasm

Until now, sex has failed to take advantage of the innate agility of fingers, and nobody has ever tried to explain the concept of the "erogenous brain" or a method for developing "erogenous routes." Ancient treatises on sex, the original "how-to" manuals such as the Indian *Kama Sutra* or the Chinese *Fangzhongshu*, don't go into detail on these subjects.

Yes, I'm saying that thanks to me, we at last have a sexual theory capable of breaking the seal on hidden female sensuality for the first time in human history.

I have helped more than a thousand women enter zones of sensuality that they had never experienced before. The technique that's the foundation of my unique method is called the "Adam Touch," which I shall describe now. The Adam Touch is not simply a way of making a woman reach orgasm. The biggest reason the Adam Touch has been praised as "unbelievable" by the women who have experienced it lies in its ability to dramatically alter a woman's sexual constitution, causing her to become more sensitive. Although it may sound like it requires some difficult, complicated maneuver, it's actually quite simple and can be performed by anyone who gets the knack.

So let's get right to it. Imagining that your stomach or thigh is a woman's body, move your fingers as follows. First, hold your hand horizontally so your palm is roughly one and a half inches from your skin, and let the tips of your fingers fall on your skin in a relaxed state. This is the basic hand shape for performing the Adam Touch. The important thing here is the "tactile pressure" of your fingers on the skin. It might help to imagine a thin film between the skin and the tips of your fingers. The tactile pressure is so light that it's almost as though your fingers aren't touching the skin, and it is this almost imperceptible pressure that transmits exactly the right amount of stimulus to your partner's erogenous zones.

The basic motion of the fingers is elliptical. For a large surface like a woman's back, move your fingers slowly in a large elliptical motion. For a medium-sized surface, such as the lower back or buttocks, use a slightly smaller motion, and for a small area, such as the palm of the hand or the top of the foot, use a small elliptical motion with just two or three fingers. There are two reasons for using an elliptical motion. First, women by nature are put at ease by regular, repeating motions. This has a relaxing effect that prepares women for greater sensitivity by putting them in a tranquil state of mind filled with feelings of peace, comfort, and trust. Second, your partner can anticipate the path traced by your fingers. This expectation, her knowing what spot of her body will be touched next, is effective in opening up her erogenous zones.

There are two basic rules you must follow when performing the elliptical motion. The first is to maintain the even spacing among your fingers. Erotic stories are filled with descriptions of supposedly dexterous fondling in which each finger wriggles "as though it were a living thing with a mind of its own." A serious misconception. It

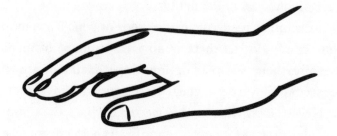

The Adam Touch

might work for a magician, but certainly not for a sexual technician. The routes to a woman's erogenous zones are opened by the continuous reception of very fine stimulus. Wiggling your fingers around will spoil the consistency of the tactile pressure, making it impossible to provide optimum stimulus in a stable manner. The first step towards mastering the Adam Touch is to make the basic hand shape I just described second nature. If you try it, you will see that although it sounds easy, it's actually pretty difficult to keep your fingers aligned. On the other hand, if you focus too much on not moving your fingertips, your entire hand will get too rigid. The result is like riding over a bumpy road on a bicycle with too much air in the tires. In order to successfully trace your fingers smoothly over the fine hills and valleys of your partner's skin while maintaining that barely perceptible tactile pressure, you have to release the tension from your fingers and achieve a certain amount of flexibility.

The other basic rule is the speed at which you move your hand. Just as there is an ideal amount of tactile pressure, there is also an optimum speed: about one inch per second. If you try it, you will see how slow this actually is. Nevertheless, this is the speed at which the almost teasingly slow movement of your fingers perfectly matches the female body's mechanism for recognizing physical stimulus as sexually pleasurable. And, like the rule about keeping your fingertips still, maintaining a speed of one inch per second can be extremely difficult for beginners. If the Adam Touch is administered accurately, however, your partner's body will begin to grow more sensitive. The erogenous routes gradually open up, and the sensual motor hidden deep within her body starts to run. This is the moment when the female body reclaims the erotic physical expression written into its DNA. Needless to say, there is not a man alive who is not aroused by a woman reacting viscerally to his stimulation, which is why it is difficult for your brain, once aroused, to maintain that speed limit. Most of the students at my school experience this at least once, almost always speeding up the motion of their hand. However, you're no longer performing the Adam Touch if you break this speed limit. Having lost its supply of optimum stimulus, the woman's erogenous brain will immediately cool down in inverse proportion to the man's hasty excitement.

Light touch with all five fingers, maintaining an elliptical motion at one inch per second, while making sure to keep the fingers from wiggling: as words on a page it appears simple, but there are many hurdles to overcome on the road to mastery of this technique. You must maintain the passion of the moment without tensing your hand. You have to hold yourself back from trying to elicit an immediate sensual reaction. Finally, you must be able to achieve just the right tactile pressure and absolute speed. This all requires a lot of practice.

There also exists another aspect of the Adam Touch apart from the specific rules I've discussed so far—namely, the "sexual energy" created by your fingers.

Consider the basic hand shape one more time. There is about an inch between the palm of your hand and the skin, and this space has a meaning. Can you guess what it is? Put the palm of your right hand on the top of your left hand so that the two hands are flat against each other. You don't feel anything other than your hand, right? Now try making the basic hand shape of the Adam Touch, and put your right hand on your left hand again. Can you feel the difference? Unlike before, you should now sense a kind of warm tingling. This is sexual energy, and it is an aspect of the *ki* (or *chi* as it's known in Chinese) energy commonly discussed in Asian martial arts. There is a very powerful pressure point in the middle of the palm of your hand that emits this energy. When out on a date, women like to hold their partner's hand. If you ask them why, they say that it makes them "feel loved." As it turns out, they feel that way because by overlapping these two pressure points, one person's *ki* blends with the other person's *ki*. The more sexually aroused you are, the more *ki* flows out. The human body sure is an amazing thing, isn't it?

But back to the topic at hand. The basic hand shape of the Adam Touch is the shape that allows the greatest generation of *ki* from the fingers, too. The synergy created by combining the fine physical stimulus of your fingers with the sexual energy they are generating is the ultimate way to turn your partner's body into one complete, uninterrupted erogenous zone.

One more note. The direction you move your hand should be clockwise, whether you are right-handed or left-handed.

Vibration as Stimulus

Most men would be surprised to hear that women's bodies are as sensitive to vibration as they are to friction. People tend to view the world through the prism of their own experience. Few are the men who have ever experienced pleasure from vibration. Accordingly, there are even fewer men who have applied vibration to stimulate their partners.

Men tend to think that the way to give a woman

pleasure is through friction, based on their own experience of rubbing their penis during masturbation. Granted, there are probably some men who have used vibrators on their partners, and vibrators can certainly apply stimulus to a very small area (the clitoris) in order to bring about a rapid orgasm. But vibrators only provide superficial vibration to the skin, and the stimulus is mechanical and often overwhelming. If women get used to achieving orgasm through this kind of stimulus, they will gradually become desensitized to their own sexual potential, which is a very dangerous thing.

The vibration I have in mind is produced by her partner's hand and fingers. I'm talking about a groundbreaking method which brings to life the latent erogenous zones in a woman's body by delivering deep interior stimulus, to areas such as the uterus, rather than just applying vibration to the outside of the body.

The method is called "Vibration Stimulus." This technique is a pillar of the Adam Technique, forming a pair with the Adam Touch.

I learned how sensitive women are to vibration when I started looking at the erogenous zones surrounding a woman's genitalia, centered on the uterus, as a single unit. Briefly, it's the entire area of a woman's body covered by her panties, which I refer to as the "mass-orgasm zone." My research has shown that applying vibration to any point in this area allows pleasure from the stimulus to reach all other parts. The reason for this is that there are groups of nerves located behind the pubic bone and behind the sacrum (a shield-shaped bone at the base of the spine to which the tail bone is connected). The vibration travels via these nerves to the erogenous brain, and the pleasure signals are fed back. This fact also proves that the various erogenous zones in a woman's body don't exist independently of each other, but rather work closely in unison through the erogenous brain. When the clitoris is stimulated with a vibrator, it is just the clitoris that feels pleasure; if you apply vibration to the pubic bone with the base of your hand, the pleasure is transmitted to the entire area, including the clitoris. No matter how vigorously you stimulate your partner's clitoris with your tongue, she will not experience this deeper pleasure, simply because the approach is wrong—in other words, men have always used methods on their partners which apply mainly to men.

At least, that is how I try to explain it to men who need to know the theory behind the method. It's a pleasure men will never know, so it can be a hard concept to grasp. But if you trust the results of my research and perform the method I describe below on your girlfriend or wife, she will experience unprecedented pleasure that will make her happy to be alive, and you will feel the power of vibration and the mysteries of the female body through your partner's reaction. It will be sexier and more erotic than anything you have seen before.

So, let's get to the description of the technique, and the erogenous zones where it is most effective. There are four basic caressing methods. We'll look at them in order.

1. Vibration with the Fingers

With your palm horizontal, bend your middle and ring fingers so they are vertical. Place the fingertips against the site you are going to vibrate and apply rhythmic vibration. The point isn't to vibrate just the surface, but rather to use the weight of your hand to press your fingertips about half an inch in from the skin and transmit the vibration to the very center of your partner's body, as it were. This method is suited to stimulation of relatively soft areas of the body, such as the breasts, the abdomen, the buttocks, the perineum, and so on.

It's particularly effective on the breasts. It's not a very well-known fact, but the area of the pectoral muscles located in a roughly two-inch-wide band going from the nipple to the side of the thorax (on both the left and right sides) is an amazing hidden erogenous zone. Vibrate the areas with a fast rhythm. The breasts, which only elicit a modest reaction when massaged, become a much more powerful erogenous zone this way.

2. Vibration with the Palm

Place the fleshy base of your hand against the site to apply vibration to it and wave your hand back and forth (like waving goodbye). This is effective when applied to areas in the mass-orgasm zone, such as the pubic bone and the tail bone.

3. Vibration with the Tips of the Fingers

With the fleshy part of the top joint of the index and middle fingers, apply small vibrations to the erogenous zones inside the vagina. This is an effective method when used on the G-spot, discussed later. Remember, though: do not scratch the skin inside the vagina with your fingers. You must place your fingers against one point, and apply the vibration there.

4. Vibration with the Penis

In this method, you do not insert your penis and thrust, but rather insert your penis deep into the vagina, pressing the opening of the vagina hard against your body. In this position, press the head of your penis against the vaginal wall, creating pressure, and move your hips so as to transmit vibration to the vagina. This will give your partner a completely different kind of pleasure than thrusting your penis in and out. This is the perfect technique for stimulating the A-spot, discussed below.

The real meaning of the importance of vibration is to augment friction with vibration, which raises the level of pleasure exponentially.

Stimulating the Hair Brings Pleasure

Few men would doubt the statement that "the stronger the stimulus, the greater the pleasure," but as a matter of fact, there is very little truth to that. Not only is the misconception one of the main factors preventing many women from experiencing orgasm, but the rough treatment causes pain and even injury to their genitalia. Such experiences can be traumatic and are a factor in causing women to go off sex altogether.

Women experience stimulus as pleasurable not on the skin of their erogenous zones, but in their brain, which receives the signals of that stimulus. Women with a high level of sensitivity in fact have a so-called "erogenous brain" that is very sensitive. If you understand this female sexual mechanism, you will automatically know what kind of stimulus is appropriate. And yes, the answer is very gentle, not strong. The principle at work here might become clearer in the context of taste. Eating strongly seasoned food on a daily basis desensitizes your tongue, and you will no longer be able to distinguish the flavor of the actual ingredients. Women's sexual sensitivity is the same. Over-seasoning (= strong stimulus) desensitizes a woman's erogenous brain and is therefore unwise. Just as loading your food down with sugar or mustard stops you from enjoying the true flavor, over-stimulating your partner makes good sex impossible.

So, what should you do to sensitize sexual receptivity? Going back to the taste example, you would gradually accustom your tongue to more subtle flavors. This may seem like a roundabout way of doing things to men used to believing that "the greater the stimulus, the greater the pleasure," but getting your partner's sexual sensitivity accustomed to very gentle stimulus is the only way to take her body to the next level of receptivity.

If you have trouble believing me, then try this: next time you stimulate your partner's clitoris, use ten percent less force than usual, and be sure not to increase the pressure even after your partner begins reacting. Keep it as gentle as at the beginning. A woman used to strong stimulus might not know what to make of it at first, since not just men, but women, too, have become used to junk sex. Maintain that gentleness. It might take longer for your partner to climax, but when she does, it will be at a much higher level than she could reach with strong stimulus. You'll see the truth of what I'm saying when it happens. Ask your partner about the experience afterwards. I can guarantee she will tell you that she prefers the new method. Providing gentle stimulation for a long period of time doesn't just give your partner the kind of pleasure that fulfills her physical cravings but allows her to experience the spiritual contentment of being loved by her man. This is the true nature of sex, which has unfortunately fallen by the wayside in our modern, junk-sex society.

It is necessary to fine-tune the stimulus in order to bring out the full potential of female sexual sensitivity. The best way to do this is to stroke your partner's hair. Try stroking your own hair, the way you would gently stroke a pet. Do you feel something? You can sense the touch, even though there are no nerve endings in hair. This is because the stimulus to the hair travels to the roots. Now try touching one of your nails. Again, there are no nerve endings in your nails, but you still feel the touch. This is the very gentle touch I'm trying to get you to use. Recall for a second how you stimulate your partner. Do you see how you've been using excessive force? Grabbing your partner's breasts, sucking on her nipples, violently rubbing her clitoris... The things the average man does to his partner without thinking are only designed to satisfy *his* urges and hardly even deserve the name "stimulus."

"Well begun is half-done" goes the old adage, and the same applies to sex. If you want to make your partner very receptive to sex, start by stroking her hair. Gently, lovingly stroking your partner's hair allows you to fine-tune her erogenous brain's sensitivity to finer stimulus. You will undoubtedly be surprised by how different her reaction is afterward.

The Face is a Treasure Trove of Erogenous Zones

I mentioned that the first switch which acts as a standard in Slow Sex is hair (the roots of the hair). Receiving the very fine stimulus applied to the roots of the hair causes the sensors in your partner's erogenous brain to adjust to fainter signals, allowing her to recognize stimuli that she previously couldn't distinguish as pleasure. In other words, she becomes more sensitive. However, you have done nothing more than fine-tune her sensors by stroking her hair. Like a brand-new radio station, you have a long way before accumulating the know-how and content to satisfy your listeners.

To go beyond this stage full of unknowns and further develop yourself, stimulus to the face is very effective. Most men, unfortunately, are not aware of this, but it is no exaggeration to call the face a "treasure trove of erogenous zones"—that's how many erogenous zones are packed onto the facial surface. When picking romantic or sexual partners, most men are very picky about a woman's facial features—liking one woman for her big eyes, rejecting another for her big nose—but when it comes to sex, they completely ignore the face. It doesn't make a lot of sense, but it's true nonetheless.

I'll digress a bit here, but upon hearing that women's bodies are one big erogenous zone from head to toe, some men yell "Eureka!" and proceed to perform enthusiastic cunnilingus with a certain self-intoxication. In other words, even when they learn that a woman's body is one big erogenous zone, they are completely unable to put to use that undisputable fact, unable to liberate themselves from the fixed idea that women feel pleasure in certain areas but not in others. And the face is one of those places that men simply don't believe women derive pleasure from being stimulated.

What a waste! The face is one of the most sensitive erogenous zones. The Adam Touch is particularly effective there, and it is ideal for helping your partner's body learn once and for all how great fine stimulation is, as you move from stroking her hair to stimulating her face.

The surfaces of the cheeks, the line of the jaw, and the lips and the area around them are particularly sensitive. Using either your index and middle fingers or your middle and ring fingers, apply the Adam Touch gently to these areas. Not only will your partner feel good, she will feel your love, increasing her arousal and raising the sensitivity of her erogenous brain.

The Interplay of *Ki* from Kissing

Nothing beats getting a good start, and in sex, kissing is key. I wrote earlier that sex is the interplay of sexual energy, and kissing is the first encounter of your and your partner's sexual energies because it is the first contact between your vital essences. Or at least, that's how it should be. In reality, junk sex reduces sex to the rapid attainment of orgasm, reducing the very value of the act. One of the major causes of this is the short shrift modern couples give to kissing. Think of your own sexual experiences. Kissing is supposed to be meaningful and to play an important role in creating a good sexual experience, but it has probably become routine, something to get over with before the act itself. Am I right?

Teaching my students, one thing I'm confronted with is the high number of men who don't give a thought to anything but pure technique, including the Adam Touch. Even though I'm imparting to my students knowledge that amounts to a trade secret—"exquisite digital stimulus and the sexual energy radiated create amazing synergy"—they focus only on moving their fingers and completely forget the sexual energy part of the equation, which is so vital. When you say *ki*, people tend to imagine some kind of inscrutable magic, but it's actually not that complicated. *Ki* basically works in conjunction with your feelings and thoughts. All you have to do is be conscious of your feelings of love for your partner when you have sex with her, and the *ki* will naturally come. Put like that, even a beginner can understand the principle.

Don't underestimate yourself. Just because you can't

see something doesn't mean it's beyond your ken. Believe in the power of your own *ki*. Believing in the existence of your *ki* and maintaining an awareness of the *ki* you are producing—even if it is invisible—helps you amplify its power, directly leading to activation of your partner's erogenous brain.

Back to kissing. If you want to have mind-blowing sex, an amazing union of desire and flesh that takes your partner to a deeper world of sensuality and earth-shattering climax, then don't overlook kissing. Make an effort to lift kissing back up from its devalued state. To this end, I will give you a valuable tip: when your and your partner's lips meet, make a conscious effort to feel the softness of her lips in the deepest part of your brain, in an emotionally moving and uplifting manner. This may sound a bit philosophical, but the ideal kiss is one that you enjoy through profound sensitivity. Enriching your sensitivity is the first step to gaining a reputation for being a good kisser and will increase the power of your *ki* before you know it.

In terms of actual technique, kissing is best thought of as stimulation of your partner's lips and tongue with your own lips and tongue. I mentioned already that a common misconception among men is that women respond to more aggressive stimulation; not surprisingly, many men think that if they vigorously jam their tongue down their partner's throat, she will get aroused. It would be great if your partner

is as aroused as you are and lustily devours your tongue,
and so on, but we've all had the uncomfortable experience
of putting our tongue in our partner's mouth only to be
greeted by clenched jaws, hesitance, and awkward silence.
This is because during the kissing stage leading up to
sex, women in general desire the kind of beautiful and
passionate embraces they see in movies. This is another
reason I say that a deep sensitivity is needed. Honestly,
men have to create a beautiful, romantic mood, hinting at
beautiful, romantic sex, even if they have to act a little bit.
Your partner wants to feel the spark of your first kiss, even
if it's your hundredth.

The Adam G-Spot—the Super Erogenous Zone

Let's start by accurately locating the G-spot.

1. With your partner lying on her back, slowly insert
your index and middle fingers into her vagina, with
the palm of your hand facing up.

2. With your fingers fully inserted, bend them at
the second joint, and press the pads of your fingers
against the pubic bone.

When you do this, your fingers are touching the
correct location of the G-spot. If you do not bend your

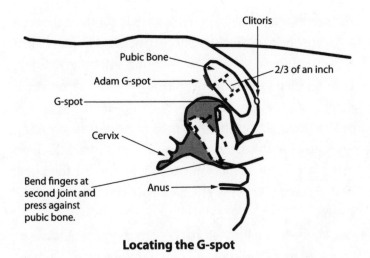

Locating the G-spot

fingers in the direction of the pubic bone, you will not reach the G-spot. This is why books that purport to teach you sexual positions that make it possible to stimulate the G-spot with your penis are full of nonsense. (Unless your penis bends at a right angle...) Descriptions of the location of the G-spot that tell you it is the area of rough skin you feel when you put your fingers one or two inches straight in are also incorrect.

If you follow steps one and two, you should be able to locate the G-spot fairly easily. The male students at my school find it the first time about 70% of the time. The problem is how to stimulate it. Getting the knack takes some time. My students only get the stimulation right the first time about half the time.

This is how it's done. With the two fingers inserted

and bent at the second joint as described above, wave your fingertips back and forth one or two inches. The movement of your fingers should be bending, then extending, bending, then extending, over and over. As a result you'll be applying pressure to the G-spot with the fleshy part of the first joint of your fingers, then releasing the pressure, and repeating this over and over at short intervals in an "on/off" type of motion to cause vibration in the pubic bone. This is the most effective way of stimulating the G-spot.

Many of you have probably seen pornographic actors jamming their fingers in and out of the actresses' vaginas, scraping the vaginal walls. This is absolutely the wrong thing to do, and should not be done, due to the risk of injury to the vaginal walls. In contrast, the method I just described involves simply repeating a motion of applying pressure and releasing pressure. No matter how fast you do it, there's no risk of injury to the vaginal walls. In fact, the faster you move your fingers, the greater the vibration effect, which increases the stimulation. I developed this method through extensive research with the cooperation of many women. To repeat, the G-spot is an erogenous zone capable of giving a woman pleasure only if you cause vibration in the pubic bone as well, by bending your fingers and pressing them against the pubic bone. Forget all the useless information you've gotten from other sex manuals. Wipe the slate clean, and remember only the description

I just gave.

Now we can get to the heart of the matter. As it turns out, during the course of my research into the G-spot, I discovered an erogenous zone that blows the G-spot out of the water—a super erogenous zone which I have christened the "Adam G-spot" to differentiate it from the conventional G-spot.

It is located about two-thirds of an inch "deeper" than the regular G-spot, deeper in the sense that, with your partner lying on her back, it's about two-thirds of an inch farther up along the pubic bone. In other words, to reach it you have to put your fingers about two-thirds of an inch further in than the position reached by your fingers when they are bent at the second joint (how you reach the conventional G-spot). To do this, you have to unbend your fingers. The method of stimulation is the same as before, but instead of bending and extending your fingers at the second joint, the fulcrum for the on/off motion is now the third joint (i.e., the knuckle).

By moving the locus of stimulus a mere two-thirds of an inch or so, you are able to deliver many more times the pleasure. In fact, the pleasure is on such a different order of magnitude that the sensation is too much for some women, so you should start by stimulating the G-spot first to get your partner used to the pleasure before going on to the next step. If performed properly on your partner, she will scream with pleasure, no matter how quiet or retiring

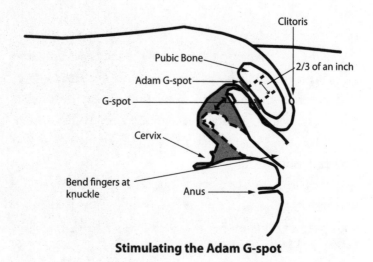

Stimulating the Adam G-spot

she may ordinarily be. I guarantee that you will witness the beauty of your partner reacting more sensually and vocally than ever before.

The Amazing T-Spot

The T-spot is another erogenous zone I discovered in the vagina. The "T" in "T-spot" stands for Tokunaga. I named it this just the way the G-spot is named after the scientist who found it. Let's take a look at where it's located and how to stimulate it.

The T-spot is found in what is called the *paries anterior vaginae*, or the anterior wall of the vagina, which is between the uterus and the pubic bone. Have your partner lie on

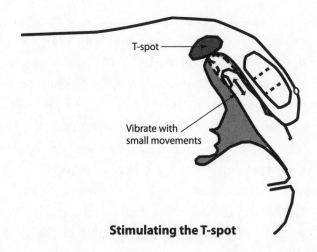

T-spot

Vibrate with
small movements

Stimulating the T-spot

her side and bend her left leg ninety degrees. Slide your
fingers into your partner's vagina parallel to the pubic
bone. The area they touch when they can go no further is
the T-spot.

You should use your index and middle fingers, with
the two fingers extended straight, as though you were
making a gun shape with your hand. This is the basic
shape.

The T-spot is stimulated as follows. First, make sure
that your fingers, the back of your hand, and your forearm
form a single straight line. With the tips of your fingers
pressed against the T-spot, apply vibration by moving your
fingers in and out of the vagina, thrusting them against
the T-spot, but not in a piston-like motion. There should
be no friction between the skin of your fingers and the skin

of the vaginal wall. Your fingers should be pressed firmly against the T-spot as you move your fingers in and out very slightly, creating vibration.

It is not easy to compare the level of pleasure derived from the T-spot and the G-spot, but there are women who say the T-spot feels better. One woman described the pleasure as "a bolt of lightning shooting from my cervix right into my brain." In other words, this is a hand technique that can literally blow your partner's mind.

That's how effective this method of stimulation is, and in terms of technique, it is easier than the G-spot or the Adam G-spot. Introduce your partner to a world of pleasure she has never experienced through ordinary penetrative sex.

The A-Spot—a Power Source of Pleasure

With the G-spot and the T-spot, vibration is the most effective stimulus, and this applies to all erogenous zones in the vagina.

I will now discuss a stimulation method using the penis, applying the concept of stimulation by vibration.

The spot to stimulate is called the A-spot (after the "A" in Adam) and is located where the head of your penis touches when you insert it into your partner's vagina. When women say that their partner's penis hits

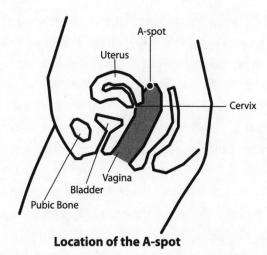

Location of the A-spot

their cervix, what they mean is the A-spot, and not the cervix (the mouth of the uterus). Until now nobody has ever realized that it is an erogenous zone, so nobody ever bothered finding out how to stimulate it properly. This is a case of simple ignorance, but it speaks volumes to the importance of correct knowledge and awareness in sex.

This is particularly true of the A-spot, which does not require any kind of complicated techniques to stimulate. Anyone can give their partner pleasure as long as they know that the A-spot is an erogenous zone and that vibration is the best way to stimulate it.

And this is how it's done.

Insert your penis as far as it will go, and it will automatically hit the A-spot. Without moving—that is, with your and your partner's lower abdomens pressed tightly against each other—apply pressure to the A-spot with your penis. Make a very small thrusting motion with your hips, transmitting the vibration from the tip of your penis to the A-spot. Remember, you only want to create vibration, not actually move your penis in and out of the vagina (i.e., creating friction). The A-spot is a very sensitive pressure point. You could almost call it the "power source of pleasure." With the right amount of vibration, it will deliver explosive impact. In fact, I have used this technique to help many women climax who say they have never had a vaginal orgasm. This technique is also suited to men who have a tendency to ejaculate quickly, since no thrusting, or skin-on-skin friction, is involved, allowing you to increase the amount of time spent in intimate pleasure between you and your partner.

Breaking Taboos, Building Trust

It goes without saying, but the biggest prerequisite for enjoying sex is liberating yourself. You can find the true freedom afforded by sex only by opening yourself up to your partner and together creating an unrestrained world where you have no secrets from each other. The reality, however, is that women's feelings of shame and taboos regarding sex stand as significant obstacles before you.

Men must help their partners overcome their feelings

of shame and release them from the taboos that make up their views of sex. It's not as easy as it sounds. Your partner will likely put up quite a bit of resistance, putting to you, for instance, "What do you know about how women feel about sex?" using the sex difference as a sort of defense. Don't be afraid, though. Men and women share an erogenous zone that is a source of shame and taboos for both sexes: the anus.

For women, the anus—the very locus of defecation!—is the one place on their body they don't want to show anyone. And not just women. Feelings of shame and a sense of taboo surrounding the anus are very strong in men, too. On the other hand, releasing yourself from anal taboos can be the quickest short cut to self-liberation. Liberating yourself from taboos regarding the anus is good for more than just getting rid of taboos. It's a little known fact that the anus is an erogenous zone more sensitive than a woman's nipples. It is worth discovering this hidden gem to experience one of the finer delicacies sex has to offer.

Words like "perverse" and "kinky" have a negative image, but what is sex, after all? It's a perverse and kinky desire to achieve pleasure with your partner. The healthiest way to look at sex is to see that in the very private space of two people in love, there can be no "perversity" or "kink." Change your approach altogether, and try regarding anal stimulation as something fun you and your partner can perform to strengthen the bonds that hold you together.

Your sex life will change drastically if you succeed in creating a relationship in which you and your partner can share the unique pleasure of oral-anal stimulation. Indeed, all your past feelings of shame and taboo will become fodder for greater excitement and arousal.

The first step in convincing your partner to do this is for you, the man, to take the initiative and ask her to orally stimulate your anus. The best time to do this is during fellatio. Don't be shy or coy. Just come out and ask her to do it. Most women will give it a try. When you use your own body to demonstrate to your partner how great an erogenous zone the anus can be, her feelings of shame will gradually break down. The next step is to return the favor when you are performing cunnilingus on your partner, making sure she is receptive to the act. Be as gentle as possible the first time. Some women will react badly, no matter how gently you may do it, though. In that case, stop immediately, and play it down with a joke—"Oops, wrong hole!" You must never force your partner to do something she doesn't want to do. But don't forget that as an erogenous zone, the anus gives more pleasure than the nipples. Don't give up too easily, and you will succeed in opening the door to new pleasures for your partner.

Once you and your partner are comfortable with oral-anal stimulation, you are ready to go to the next level—manual penetration of the anus. To do this, you will need two things: latex gloves (available at most pharmacies) and massage oil (which you can find at stores like The Body Shop). There are hygienic reasons for using gloves, but they are also good for inducing a sense of security on that point.

The best position is either lying on the back with the legs spread and the knees back (the legs forming an "M"), or on all fours. Use your middle finger for insertion. Thoroughly lubricate your middle finger and the area around the anus with the massage oil. Start by gently massaging the anus with your finger before insertion. Once your partner is comfortable with this and some of the tension in the anus itself has dissipated, insert your finger up to the first joint. Once in, pull it out slowly. Repeat this in-and-out motion many times, without rushing. When you judge the time is right, next insert your finger up to the second joint. Repeat the in-and-out motion again, as before. The skin of the anus tears easily, so use a very slow and gentle rhythm. The effect is not changed by inserting your finger deeper than the second joint, so stop at the second joint.

Once you have mastered insertion, the second step is to introduce vibration stimulus. Instead of the in-and-out motion, keep your finger inserted and move it up and down and left and right. You will be able to arouse your partner by imparting the vibration throughout the "mass-orgasm zone." You can also stimulate your partner's clitoris with your thumb while stimulating her anus. The combined effect is powerful, so give it a try.

Here are two more techniques that are effective. When you insert your finger straight in, it will hit a rigid protrusion. That's the cervix. Apply vibration with the tip of your finger using a motion like that of a bird pecking the ground.

The other technique is stimulation of the G-spot from inside the anus. If you insert your finger as far as you can and bend it towards the pubic bone, it will hit the G-spot. Apply vibration, and you will achieve a "double-punch" of simultaneous G-spot and anal stimulation. This is a special technique that will have your partner screaming with pleasure.

Once you have broken down the taboos, feel free to explore the new world of sensuality that has opened up to you.

A New Position for Starting

Often, intercourse (penetration) begins in the missionary position.

The problem with this, as I described in Chapter One, is that the missionary position is capable of making even ordinary men ejaculate prematurely—it's the "premature ejaculation" position. Thus it's a big problem that initiating intercourse in the missionary position has become so normal, without anyone even giving it a second thought. Many of the ideas we have about sex are, in fact, mistaken.

If our concern is simply to enable men to hold out longer before ejaculation, then it should suffice for the man to lie on his back, suppressing arousal by bringing the relaxing effects of the parasympathetic nervous system to the fore. The problem with this is that it's not always realistic to expect a woman to agree to be on top at the beginning. What I recommend, therefore, is a position (which I call "modified missionary") in which you and your partner are facing each other, like in the missionary position, but with the man's upper body raised so that it is nearly perpendicular to the bed surface. This simple change alters the predicament of the penis completely. By putting your upper body in a vertical position, you are putting the sympathetic nervous system, which promotes arousal, and the parasympathetic nervous system, which suppresses arousal, into a neutral state. This suppresses excess arousal even in men who do not have a lot of confidence in their ability to hold out, allowing them to control the timing of their ejaculation to a certain degree. If you try out the modified missionary position, you'll immediately know what I am talking about. In addition, by slightly impeding the movement of your hips, this position stops you from overdoing it down there. Greater self-confidence will change the way you have sex and give you a greater sense of your own potential.

Sitting is the New Standard Position

More than anything, a woman wants to feel that her partner loves her. As such, she strongly desires to feel his body pressed against hers. Women have a tendency to pull closer to their partners the greater their arousal during sex and the better it feels. This can be a problem if you've just initiated intercourse as described above, with your upper body vertical, and your partner tries to pull you closer (i.e., down towards her), forcing you into "premature ejaculation" mode and bringing you back to square one.

But not to worry—there is a well-known position capable of satisfying both the man's desire to extend his endurance and the woman's desire to feel the loving sensation of her partner's body against hers. The position is known as "sitting."

In the sitting position, the man's upper body is upright, so he can relax as his arousal is suppressed, and the movement of his hips is limited, too, making it easier to hold off ejaculation. On the woman's part, she can press her body against her partner's and feel that sense of togetherness she craves. Each partner is supporting the other's body, which reduces fatigue. In addition, since your faces are close to each other, you can kiss and talk to your heart's content. In many respects, sitting is the ideal position for enjoying Slow Sex.

Incidentally, the *Kama Sutra*, the ancient Indian guide

to sex, calls the sitting position the "normal position," describing it as the default standard. This just goes to show how different the culture of sex was in ancient India, where love-making was assumed to be best when unhurried.

Truly overcoming premature ejaculation requires a great deal of time and patience. Learning the pros and cons of various positions makes longer love-making possible—and that's the essence of Slow Sex, after all! If you are one of the many men who has never experienced the interaction of your and your partner's sexual energies because there has been too little time between penetration and ejaculation, then I highly recommend changing your main position from the missionary position to the sitting one. Experience the joy of your sexual energies interacting.

Thirty Minutes of Loveplay, Thirty Minutes of Intercourse

The fundamental rule of Slow Sex is "forget the clock and have fun." The problem with the word "foreplay" is that it presumes a kind of separation between "sex designed to bring about orgasm" and "sex not designed to bring about orgasm." By eliminating the notion of time (or limits), you can bring out the full potential of your partner's erogenous brain, letting her relax in mind and body. In other words, forgetting the clock means removing upper limits on pleasure and arousal, allowing your partner to show her true, unconcealed self in all her primordial sensuality.

The reality is that there are limits on time, however. You're tired and need to get to sleep early, you've got a meeting first thing in the morning, you're afraid the kids will wake up... Many and various are the ways our lives are controlled by the clock. Nonetheless, when it comes to sex, it is important to tell yourself that you have all the time in the world, plenty of time for both you and your partner to be satisfied.

Therefore, while including time in the equation is contrary to the spirit of the method, I will discuss this issue in terms of a rule of thumb for Slow Sex beginners who have picked up this book.

The basic rule of thumb: "thirty minutes of loveplay and thirty minutes of intercourse." While the current average of fifteen minutes of foreplay and five minutes of intercourse may suffice for a man to reach orgasm, there is no way a woman can even reach full arousal within that time frame. You must go beyond it.

Note that thirty minutes of loveplay doesn't include kissing, fellatio, or other stimulus your partner gives you. Thirty minutes is the minimum amount of time needed for you to stimulate your partner using the Adam Touch and other techniques. For Slow Sex beginners, this may seem like a long time, but once you've correctly mastered the Adam Touch imparted in these pages, your partner will show you an erotic and sensual side of herself that you have never seen before. You'll soon realize how short thirty minutes is. Even men who tend to ejaculate prematurely will be able to hold out with ease as long as they remember that the basic positions are the modified missionary and sitting positions, and that sex is more than just thrusting their pelvis. Once you start to feel that the initial goal of "thirty minutes of loveplay, thirty minutes of intercourse" is not such a long time, you will have graduated the beginner course. Your next goal: "one hour of loveplay, and endless intercourse."

That's where Slow Sex begins.

"Long Sex" and Your View of Sex

As I've mentioned many times already, the true essence of sex is the "interaction of sexual energies."

As the sexual energies you and your partner generate mixes and circulates throughout your bodies, the total sexual energy becomes greater than the sum of its parts. Your partner's erogenous brain matures and becomes more and more sensitive, and sexual energy grows at an exponential rate.

What is the one thing in sex you can do to best promote the interaction of sexual energy? The answer is intercourse (penetration). Sexual energy interacts just by holding hands and kissing, but it goes without saying that intercourse, which can aptly be compared to "putting the plug in the socket," is the most efficient and rational way to cause sexual energies to interact. The longer the period of time the plug is in and you're "turned on," the greater the amount of sexual energy produced. It's obvious.

In this section I want to go into a bit of detail about the essence of Slow Sex—"long sex," a gateway to a level of sensuality unattainable by men who think of sex as nothing more than skin rubbing against skin.

The average amount of time I spend penetrating my partner is two hours. On hearing this, most women react by saying that that's too long, that it would wear them out. Women who have only ever experienced junk sex, with their partner penetrating them and pumping away for five minutes, imagine my two hours to be an extended version of the kind of sex they have. If that were the case, it would tire *me* out, and the woman's vagina would undoubtedly start hurting. The fact is that I don't spend the entire two hours pumping away. My partner and I enjoy the sensuality created by the interaction of our sexual energies, while at the same time experiencing the pleasure of friction from the penetration.

I just wrote "my partner and I," and this is a very important point. It is vital that the man approach sex knowing about sexual energy and intending to create an interaction in sexual energies, but, like unrequited love, the *ki* cannot mix efficiently if only one partner is aware of all this. The woman must also make an effort to enjoy this interaction of sexual energies. When both partners are on the same wavelength, intercourse goes from being something that you must complete to something you never want to stop.

Indeed, if Slow Sex is performed correctly, there is no fatigue involved. The longer the intercourse, the greater the sum of sexual energy. Fatigue? Far from it! You become more energized in your total focus on enjoying each other's bodies.

In order to ensure a smooth changing of the guard in your approach to sex, coital technique is not to be neglected. You have to revise your previous notions about penetration, which used to be centered on you and your pleasure, and see that penetration is one more way of stimulating the vagina, albeit with your penis. This alone should change the way you thrust your pelvis. The biggest misconception in sex has been that both men and women have wanted to attain orgasm early, focusing solely on high-intensity stimulus. By focusing instead on low-intensity pleasure without worrying about the time, letting your feelings and motions wander freely, you can achieve a kind of ejaculation and climax so intense that it can only be called an "explosion," thanks to your sexual energies combining and reaching a critical point.

However, if the woman doesn't have the proper awareness of the interaction of sexual energies, her erogenous brain won't fully open up, and she will only be able to recognize less intense pleasure as "weak" or "boring." If only you, who have read this book, are ready for the experience, and your partner can't understand what's going on, the sex won't be so great. Just like you, your partner must be educated about the sad fact of the spread of junk sex and its ill effects. You must impart to your partner the correct knowledge of sex you have learned from this book. If you want to take the lead as a man, you have to enlighten your partner.

Slow Sex Needs No "Warming Down"

According to books on the topic, "afterplay is more important than foreplay." I beg to differ; I've never had this "afterplay." In fact, it might be more accurate to say that afterplay is impossible.

The grand finale of Slow Sex is something close to an explosion of pleasure. The careful and scrupulous application of the Adam Touch combined with an hour or more intercourse results in the sexual energies of both partners reaching a critical point and eventually exploding. I imagine most men have occasionally experienced a relaxing fatigue after fairly satisfactory sex, but Slow

Sex culminates in something beyond compare. You're completely spent—your power indicator reads "zero." You and your partner fall into a sleep like quicksand. That's how things work with Slow Sex.

So when people describe "afterplay" like a natural addition to sex, they're missing the obvious point that making "afterplay" part of the plan right from the start just builds in the assumption that the partner will not be fully satisfied with the sex itself. People who preach the importance of "afterplay" with a knowing tone are in essence revealing the paltriness of their own techniques and understanding of sex. Nothing could be more pathetic.

Theory, Technique, and Training

Having read this far, you have undoubtedly realized to what extent commonly held concepts of sex are nothing more than misconceptions arising from male prejudice and ignorance. You are now in possession of a true understanding of how sex works and techniques to make it better. Your consciousness has been raised through acquisition of accurate knowledge, and this will continue to make your sex life evolve.

Your likelihood of bringing a woman to orgasm has undoubtedly increased. This I can guarantee.

But that's not enough. You're now only at the start

line of Slow Sex. The reason is simple: you have merely acquired the theory. In other words, you have yet to master the technique. Your task here on is to use this theory of sex as a springboard and to motivate yourself to train and master the skills required.

That's right: sex requires training.

People work hard to achieve happiness. If you want to attend a prestigious university, you study hard. If you want to be good at a sport, you practice hard. Whether it's work or a hobby, if you want to excel, you spend more time practicing, you spend money on equipment, you try to up your efficiency. Everyone knows this from experience, and everyone does it. But for whatever unfathomable reason, when it comes to sex, people's brains refuse to accept the idea of "training."

Take professional baseball players. They practice all the time to maintain their skills and to push themselves even further. Granted, they're pros, so they're born with a certain amount of talent; and yet, they run until they're sopping wet, they practice thousands or even tens of thousands of swings and more, thereby pounding the fundamentals into their bodies. It's true even in the case of someone like Ichiro Suzuki, one of the best players in the world. I doubt anyone would disagree that daily practice is the basis of first-class ability.

The most important thing for improving your technique is mastering the basics. The Adam Touch, which is the heart of the Slow Sex method, is a very simple technique. This means that anyone can mimic the shapes and motions in a very superficial manner. However, achieving just the right tactile pressure and speed to match a woman's sexual mechanism demands the highest degree of accuracy and endurance possible. You could even say that its simplicity makes it that much harder to truly master the technique. The same applies to the other techniques I've discussed. Simply learning the theory is not enough.

What you need to do now is realize that, in terms of the Slow Sex method, you are no different from a very smart college grad with zero life experience. Train until your hands acquire the knowledge that currently resides only in your brain, and you will have thoroughly mastered the fundamentals. The proof is in the practice. Shaky technique due to a lack of training won't do any good in bed. Remember well that theory, technique, and training are a trinity.

Of course, you can't practice sex the way you practice swinging a baseball bat. Pace yourself. After all, your training partner (and coach) is the woman you love. Enjoy yourselves as you follow the path to complete mastery.